WRITING FOR
PUBLICATION
IN NURSING

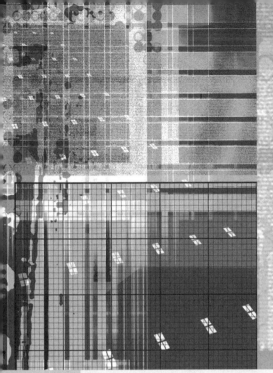

WRITING FOR
PUBLICATION
IN NURSING

Marilyn H. Oermann, PhD, RN, FAAN
Professor, College of Nursing
Wayne State University, Detroit, Michigan

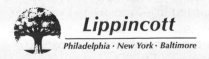
Lippincott
Philadelphia · New York · Baltimore

Acquisitions Editor: Margaret Zuccarini
Developmental Editor: Hilarie Surrena
Editorial Assistant: Helen Kogut
Senior Production Manager: Helen Ewan
Managing Editor/Production: Barbara Ryalls
Production Coordinator: Patricia McCloskey
Art Director: Carolyn O'Brien
Interior Designer: Holly Reid McLaughlin
Cover Designer: Melissa Walters
Manufacturing Manager: William Alberti
Indexer: Nancy Newman
Compositor: LWW

Library of Congress Cataloging-in-Publication Data
Oermann, Marilyn H.
    Writing for publication in nursing / Marilyn H. Oermann.
      p. ; cm.
    Includes bibliographical references and index.
    ISBN 0-7817-2555-0 (alk. paper)
     1. Nursing–Authorship. 2. Medical writing. 3. Nursing–Periodicals. I. Title.
    [DNLM: 1. Writing–Nurses' Instruction. 2. Periodicals–Nurses' Instruction. 3.
    Publishing–Nurses' Instruction. 4. Research–methods–Nurses' Instruction. WZ 345
    O29w 2001]
    RT24.O35 2001
    808'.06661–dc21
                                                                    2001029909

Care has been taken to confirm the accuracy of the information presented and to describe generally accepted practices. However, the authors, editors, and publisher are not responsible for errors or omissions or for any consequences from application of the information in this book and make no warranty, express or implied, with respect to the content of the publication.

The authors, editors, and publisher have exerted every effort to ensure that drug selection and dosage set forth in this text are in accordance with the current recommendations and practice at the time of publication. However, in view of ongoing research, changes in government regulations, and the constant flow of information relating to drug therapy and drug reactions, the reader is urged to check the package insert for each drug for any change in indications and dosage and for added warnings and precautions. This is particularly important when the recommended agent is a new or infrequently employed drug.

Some drugs and medical devices presented in this publication have Food and Drug Administration (FDA) clearance for limited use in restricted research settings. It is the responsibility of the health care provider to ascertain the FDA status of each drug or device planned for use in his or her clinical practice.

To David, Ross, and Eric

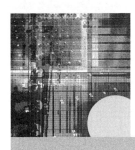

CONTRIBUTORS

CHAPTER 4
ETHICAL AND LEGAL ISSUES IN WRITING FOR PUBLICATION

Kathleen B. Gaberson, PhD, RN

Professor, Duquesne University School of Nursing
Pittsburgh, Pennsylvania

CHAPTER 15
WORLD WIDE WEB AND ELECTRONIC PUBLISHING:
Early Experiences and Future Trends

Mary Anne Rizzolo, EdD, RN, FAAN

Executive Director, Nursingcenter.com
Lippincott Williams & Wilkins
New York, New York

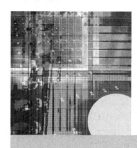

PREFACE

Writing for Publication in Nursing was prepared for beginning and experienced authors, for nurses who want to learn how to write and publish articles, and for graduate students in nursing who need to learn how to write research reports, clinical articles, and other types of articles. The book describes the process of writing, beginning with an idea, searching the literature, preparing an outline, writing a draft and revising it, and developing the final paper. How to select a journal and gear the writing to the intended audience, submit a manuscript to a journal, revise a paper and respond to reviewers, correct proofs, and carry out other steps to facilitate publication are discussed in the book. A chapter is devoted to writing research manuscripts to assist nurses in preparing their work for publication; strategies are included for developing manuscripts from theses and dissertations. Other chapters describe principles for writing clinical articles, manuscripts on professional topics and issues in nursing, philosophical and theoretical articles, case reports, and other types of papers.

The book serves as a reference for students in undergraduate nursing programs who need to learn how to write papers for courses. Many nursing programs expect students to demonstrate competency in writing as an outcome of the program. *Writing for Publication in Nursing* is a good resource for that purpose.

Writing for Publication in Nursing can be used in conjunction with the style manual in the nursing program. While style manuals direct students in preparing citations, references, tables, and figures, and guide them on other aspects of style, these manuals do not teach students the process of writing nor how to prepare a paper for publication in nursing.

The book contains many examples and resources for writing in nursing and other health fields. These resources make writing easier for both beginning and experienced authors.

Writing for publication in nursing is essential to communicate knowledge and share expertise with other nurses, inform nurses of initiatives and innovations developed for patient populations and settings, disseminate the findings of research, and advance the profession. Writing manuscripts is hard work, but the process can be simplified by understanding how to develop a manuscript and submit it for publication. Chapter 1 introduces the steps the author follows in planning, writing, and publishing manuscripts in nursing. The focus is on early writing decisions, such as generating ideas, selecting a topic, and deciding on the type of article to be written. The author evaluates if the ideas to be presented are worth writing about and are important enough to be published.

The next steps are to identify the audience to whom the manuscript will be directed and to select a journal that might be interested in publishing it. The purpose of the manuscript and how it will be developed guide the author in deciding on possible journals. The goal is to match the topic and type of manuscript with an appropriate journal and readers who would be interested in it. How to review possible journals, select an appropriate one, and write a query letter are discussed in Chapter 2. Valuable resources in this chapter include a description of Web sites of directories of journals, checklists for determining the audience and the "right" journal, and a sample query letter.

Decisions about the focus of the manuscript, audience, and journal are important early in the writing process. Another decision deals with authorship, which is discussed in Chapter 3. Authorship should be determined before beginning the writing project to avoid problems and conflict among the authors later on. Because many papers are written in groups, strategies are provided to facilitate this process, including a checklist of the responsibilities of the first author and a tracking form for group writing projects, among others.

In Chapter 4 ethical and legal issues affecting writing for publication are examined. These include justified and unjustified authorship; wasteful or duplicate publication; the submission of fraudulent, false, or fabricated data; plagiarism or misappropriation of the ideas of others; conflict of interest or competing interests among authors and peer reviewers; and protecting the rights of individuals in publications. This chapter examines these issues and offers suggestions for preventing or minimizing ethical and legal problems related to writing for publication.

The author should understand copyright principles, how to obtain permission to use copyrighted material, and issues with copyright, which also are discussed in Chapter 4. Sample permission credit lines and an example of a letter that can be used when requesting permission to reprint are included. Copyright transfer is discussed, and a sample form is provided for readers to review.

Chapter 5 prepares the author for conducting and writing a literature review for a manuscript. Although literature reviews for research studies, theses and dissertations, course work, clinical projects, and other purposes vary in the types of literature used, their comprehensiveness, and how they are summarized for the reader, the process of reviewing the literature is the same. Chapter 5 describes bibliographic databases useful for literature reviews in nursing, selecting databases to use, search strategies, analyzing and synthesizing the literature, and writing the literature review for a manuscript and other types of papers. Sample writing styles for literature reviews are included. This chapter provides many tools to help readers with their literature reviews such as a guide for analyzing nursing literature, forms for taking notes when reading nonresearch and research articles (quantitative and qualitative), and a form for summarizing the research read during the literature review. The outcome of the chapter is to develop skill in conducting literature reviews for writing papers in nursing.

Research projects are not complete until the findings are communicated to others. All too often nurses conduct important research studies but fail to disseminate the results of their work. Some nurses are not prepared for their role as an author and are unsure how to proceed. Others may believe that their work does not warrant publication, but "good" research is important to communicate to others even when the findings were not anticipated. Chapter 6 guides the author in writing research papers. The chapter begins with a discussion of how to report research using the conventional format of introduction; literature review, which may be incorporated in the introduction; methods; results; and discussion. When developing research papers for clinical journals, this format may not be explicit, but it serves as a framework for the author to use in deciding how to organize the content. Guidelines and many examples are provided for writing each part of a research paper. Discussion is included for writing qualitative research manuscripts.

Chapter 7 presents strategies for writing clinical practice, professional role, issue, philosophical and theoretical, and review articles. Other forms of writing such as case reports, editorials, book reviews, letters to the editor, and articles for consumer and nonprofessional audiences also are examined. These types of manuscripts differ in the purposes they are trying to achieve, their format, and often writing style. The last section of the chapter provides some guidelines for writing chapters and books.

Writing for publication requires careful planning, organization, and personal strategies to keep on target until the paper is completed. It can not be done haphazardly. With an outline, even if brief, and materials assembled, the author can move quickly into writing the first draft. The author should plan on revising the draft a number of times until satisfied with the final copy. Chapter 8 focuses on organizing the content, including how to develop an outline, and writing the first draft of the manuscript. In writing the first draft, the author focuses on presenting and organizing the content rather than on grammar, punctuation, spelling, and writing style.

Chapter 9 describes the steps in revising the content and organization of the paper and then revising the writing structure and style. Principles are provided for improving how the paper is written. The chapter has many valuable resources for writers including, among others, questions for revising the paper's content and organization, a list of unnecessary words often used in writing and more concise ones to replace them, and checklists for revising writing structure and style and for confirming scientific style.

Most papers written for publication in nursing include references. The references in the manuscript document the literature reviewed by the author in preparation of the paper and provide support for the ideas in it. In Chapter 10 the focus is on citing the references in the manuscript and preparing the reference list. Journals have different reference formats, and the author must prepare the references according to the journal guidelines. Most of these reference styles are based on either the name–year system or citation–sequence system. These two systems are discussed in the chapter, and examples are provided of how to cite references in the text and on the reference list using both of them.

Tables are essential when the author needs to report detailed information and numeric values. It is often clearer and more efficient to develop a table than to present the information in the text. Figures, such as graphs and charts, are valuable for demonstrating trends and patterns. For some manuscripts the author may even include an illustration of a new procedure or equipment, or a photograph of a patient. Not every manuscript, though, needs tables and figures, and whether to include them is a decision made during the drafting phase of writing the paper. Chapter 11 provides guidelines for deciding when to prepare tables and figures and how to develop them. Examples are included of different types of tables, presenting information in a table and as text when text is preferred and when a table is preferred, and figures.

At this point in the writing process, the author has completed the revisions of the content and format of the paper; has prepared the references, tables, and figures; and is ready to submit the paper to the journal. Prior to submission, there are some final responsibilities of the author to ensure that the manuscript is consistent with the journal requirements and contains all the required parts for submission. The manuscript is then ready to send to the journal for review. Chapter 12 describes the steps in preparing the final paper to submit to the journal and details associated with this submission. A sample cover letter is provided in the chapter, and a checklist is included for authors to ensure that all items are sent with the manuscript to avoid delays in its review.

Chapter 13 presents the editorial review process from the point at which the paper is received in the journal office through the final editorial decision. The roles and responsibilities of the editor, editorial board, and peer reviewers are discussed, and examples are provided of criteria used by reviewers when asked to critique a manuscript for publication. Peer review is not without issues, and some of these are examined in the chapter. Manuscripts submitted to a journal may be accepted without revision or accepted provisionally pending revision, may be returned to the author for a major revision and resubmission, or may be rejected. Each of these editorial decisions has implications for the author and how the author responds to the editor; these are presented in the chapter. Resources for readers include sample peer review forms from research, clinical, and other types of nursing journals and sample letters to send with revised manuscripts.

When the manuscript is accepted for publication, the paper moves into the publishing phase. The author has some responsibilities here, such as answering queries and correcting page proofs, but most of the work is done by the publisher of the journal or by the group or individual responsible for the publication. The manuscript is edited for clarity and consistency with the journal style and format; the copy editor more than likely will have questions about the manuscript for the author to answer. These questions, or queries, must be answered and the proofs must be reviewed, to confirm the accuracy of the content after editing and to check other details, in the time frame allowed. Chapter 14 describes the publishing process that begins with the acceptance of the paper through its publication. Publishers have different ways of handling the manuscript editing phase and forms of the manuscript that they return to the author for proofing. The publishing process is described in the chapter with the recognition that this may differ across journals.

In the final chapter information is provided on electronic publishing. Electronic publishing provides many new opportunities for nurse authors. The chapter begins with a historical perspective, discusses publishing on the Web, and examines future trends.

Many individuals have contributed to the preparation and writing of this book. The author extends a special acknowledgment to Margaret Zuccarini who recognized the need for this resource for nursing authors and students. Her enthusiasm for writing in nursing is contagious. A special thank you is extended to Nancy A. Wilmes, who is a superb librarian at Wayne State University in Detroit, Michigan. Nancy answered many of my questions and helped me gather information for Chapter 5.

Finally, a special thanks to my family, David, Ross, and Eric, who have become used to my writing and typing. Thank you for your support with this book and with my earlier ones.

Marilyn Oermann

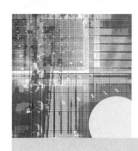

CONTENTS

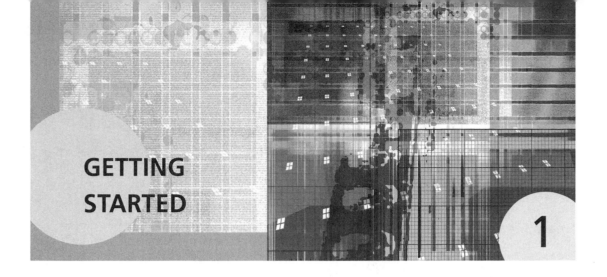

GETTING STARTED

1

Writing for publication in nursing is essential to communicate knowledge and share expertise with other nurses, inform nurses of initiatives and innovations developed for patient populations and settings, disseminate the findings of research, and advance the profession. Writing manuscripts is hard work, but the process can be simplified by understanding how to develop a manuscript and submit it for publication.

This chapter introduces the steps the author follows in planning, writing, and publishing manuscripts in nursing. The focus is on early writing decisions, such as generating ideas, selecting a topic, and deciding on the type of article to be written. These are important decisions because they direct the author in selecting potential journals, which is addressed in Chapter 2.

REASONS TO WRITE

Writing for publication is an important skill for nurses to develop. By communicating new initiatives and innovations in clinical practice, findings of research, and other ideas about nursing, nurses direct the future of their practice and advance the development of the profession. Nurses in all roles need to learn how to write for publication as a means of disseminating new knowledge for the care of patients. Writing for publication cannot be considered the responsibility of only nurses in academic settings, since clinicians have a major responsibility to describe the effectiveness of their nursing interventions and the innovations they have developed for patient care. Nurse educators, administrators, managers, and researchers have a similar responsibility: to share knowledge and ideas for the benefit of others. Writing for publication provides a durable means of communicating new knowledge and ideas to nurses and other health care providers (Ashworth, 1998).

There are five main reasons to write for publication: (1) to share ideas and expertise with other nurses; (2) to disseminate the findings of nursing research; (3) for promotion, tenure, and other personnel decisions; (4) for development of the nurse's own knowledge and skills; and (5) for personal satisfaction.

Share Ideas and Expertise

Writing for publication provides a way of sharing ideas with other nurses. Through publications, nurses are able to describe best practices; innovations developed for patients, students, and staff; and new techniques they are using in clinical practice, teaching, management, and administration. Publications keep nurses abreast of new developments in nursing.

Disseminate Research Findings

For nurses involved in research, writing for publication is an essential part of the research process. Disseminating research findings through publications is essential to contribute to the knowledge base of nursing, to provide evidence for nursing practice and ultimately use the research findings in practice, and to develop studies that build on one another. The essence of a discipline is its body of scientific knowledge, values and ethics that guide practice, and worth to society (American Association of Colleges of Nursing, 1999). In practice disciplines such as nursing, an added responsibility is the utilization of research findings in practice. Research findings can be applied to practice only if they are published and made available for use by other clinicians and nursing professionals. All too often, nurses conduct important research without disseminating the findings of these studies to others.

Meet Promotion, Tenure, and Other Job Requirements

For nursing faculty in colleges and universities, writing for publication is required for promotion, tenure, and other personnel decisions. Not all articles carry the same weight in these decisions. Typically, research papers published in refereed journals are more important than are nonresearch articles. Refereed journals use peer reviewers, or referees, to read and critique the manuscript as a basis for the acceptance decision. Although the responsibilities of peer reviewers differ with each journal, in general, peer reviewers critically read each manuscript based on predetermined criteria, identify areas for revision, and give expert opinions on the paper. With some journals, the peer reviewers also suggest possible decisions as to whether the manuscript should be accepted, revised and resubmitted, or rejected. The peer review process is discussed in Chapter 13.

The importance given to writing books and chapters varies across institutions. Nursing faculty should be aware of the weight given to different types of publications in their own institutions.

Although nurses in clinical settings are not faced with promotion and tenure decisions, writing for publication may be a requirement for job mobility and career advancement. Whether the article is data based or published in a refereed journal may be less important than writing for journals read by nurses who need this new information to guide their practice.

Expand Personal Knowledge and Skills

Another reason to write for publication is the learning gained in the process of preparing the manuscript. Rarely is the nurse able to write a manuscript without completing a thorough review of the literature. This literature review and the research that needs to be done in developing the manuscript contribute to the the author's knowledge base and understanding.

Gain Personal Satisfaction

Writing also gives the nurse a sense of personal satisfaction in sharing expertise with other nurses and contributing to the development of their practice. Considering that most professional journals do not pay authors for their manuscripts, nurses do not gain financial reward for writing an article, but they have immense personal satisfaction in seeing their name in print (McConnell, 1999).

 BARRIERS TO WRITING

Writing often is difficult, and the author may be frustrated by the time and effort needed to prepare the manuscript. Developing a publishable paper requires practice, and the more writing the author does, the easier it will be to complete a manuscript. Similar to the development of clinical skills, writing improves with practice.

Henninger and Nolan (1998) compared two group education programs for promoting publications by nurses who were novice authors. Nurses in both groups attended three monthly sessions on writing and publishing. One group received additional guidance for a year. The publication rates were similar in both groups. The authors concluded that publications by nurses who are novice authors can be facilitated by short-term guidance on how to write articles in nursing. Getting assistance in writing helps make the "work" easier.

Writer's Block

Some authors experience writer's block, which keeps them from writing. To overcome writer's block, Sheridan and Dowdney (1997) suggest that authors identify what is blocking their writing, talk with colleagues about their topic as a way of clarifying their ideas, use past writing successes to encourage current efforts, and stay with the topic until the manuscript is completed.

Lack of Understanding of How to Write for Publication

Another barrier is not knowing how to write for publication. Before beginning any manuscript, the author needs to first understand the writing and publishing processes. Often, students believe that the A+ paper they completed as a requirement in one of their nursing courses is publishable; this may or may not be true. When papers prepared for course work are submitted for publication and then rejected, the authors may become discouraged and not continue with their writing (Plawecki, 1994). Papers prepared for a course may be at a level too low for readers of a journal who have specialized knowledge and a more advanced understanding of the topic. Or, the course paper may not be in an appropriate writing style for the journal to which it was submitted. These papers may read like a thesis rather than an article (Bragadóttir, 1998). A better understanding of how to write for publication helps the author avoid situations such as these.

Lack of Time

The extensive time for preparing a manuscript is another barrier to writing. Time is needed for preliminary work such as developing the idea and reviewing the literature, for preparing the draft and rewriting it until suitable for submission, and for subsequent revisions suggested by the editor and reviewers. Time for writing is needed by all authors, novice and experienced.

Fear of Rejection

Another barrier to writing is fear of rejection (McConnell, 1999; Oermann, 1999b; Sheridan & Dowdney, 1997). In submitting a manuscript, the author is open to criticism and possible rejection; for some nurses, this is a barrier to writing for publication. Having a manuscript rejected is part of the writing process and may not be related to the quality of the writing. The manuscript may be rejected because a similar one already has been accepted, or the information in the manuscript is not new enough for publication in that particular journal. Rejections for reasons such as these do not mean that the ideas are questionable or poorly presented. Even if the manuscript is rejected because of criticisms of the research design, ideas in the manuscript, or format, the author can use this feedback as a way of learning more about the writing process, for developing writing skills further, and for revising the manuscript for submission elsewhere.

 ## PERSONAL STRATEGIES

Writing manuscripts requires setting dates for completion, using personal strategies to keep on target, meeting deadlines, and wisely using the limited time available. A manuscript can be doomed to failure if the author does not manage the time allotted for writing and completing other aspects of preparing the manuscript for submission to a journal.

Set Due Date for Completion of Manuscript

First, a due date should be set for completion of the manuscript, whether it is a journal article, a chapter in a book, a research proposal, or another writing project. The due date for completing the final copy should be realistic, considering work and personal responsibilities, and should not be altered; modifying the due date for completion of a manuscript often becomes a pattern, and the manuscript is never finished or takes too long to complete.

Divide Content into Manageable Parts With Due Dates

Second, after setting the due date for completion of the final manuscript, the author can divide the content areas into manageable parts and identify dates for completing each of these. In this way, smaller content areas are viewed as separate writing assignments with individual due dates. If the author is working from an outline, which is discussed in Chapter 8, dates can be assigned to different sections of the outline.

Third, along with dividing the manuscript into sections, each with its own due date, the author can assign due dates for completing the literature review, writing the first and subsequent drafts, preparing references, and completing other activities such as sending letters for permission to reprint.

Fourth, the author should not waiver from these due dates because with busy schedules, delays are difficult to make up later. Oermann (1999a) recommended posting the list of due dates in a prominent place.

Even with due dates, some writers have difficulty getting started and others have difficulty finishing. Viewing the manuscript in terms of smaller writing assignments and completing a few sections of the content often provide sufficient momentum and reinforcement to continue writing until the manuscript is completed.

Identify Prime Time for Writing

Authors need to identify their prime time for writing, when they are most productive and creative (Oermann, 1999a). This prime time then should be used for writing and should be guarded so that other activities do not interfere with it. Along the same line, the author should avoid interruptions and distractions during this time allotted for writing. Other times of the day may be used for activities that require less concentration, such as preparing the reference list. Fondiller (1994) recommended creating a "writing environment," which includes having a comfortable well-lit area for writing, removing distractions, writing at regular times, and having resources on hand such as style guides.

 ## STEPS IN WRITING FOR PUBLICATION

Every article written for publication begins with a planning phase; progresses to writing a draft, revising it, and submitting the final copy to the journal; and concludes with its publication. These phases, which provide a framework for the organization of the book, are discussed in more detail in subsequent chapters.

Planning Phase

Before writing the manuscript, the author proceeds through a series of steps. These steps are important to assist the author in selecting a topic that is publishable, choosing an appropriate journal with readers who are interested in the topic, and tailoring the content and format for the journal.

Identifying the Topic

The first step in the planning phase is to identify the topic or focus of the manuscript. In some cases, the focus is to present research findings or to describe the implications of a research study. The intent of other manuscripts may be to present new nursing and patient care practices, describe nursing interventions for patients with particular health problems, analyze trends and issues in practice, and present new directions in nursing management or education.

Keeping a log of ideas that might lead to a publication is one way of identifying topics to write about later. Halm (1997) recommended logging ideas into an "idea file" and looking for similarities in them to develop the manuscript.

For some manuscripts, identifying the topic is easy because the author has a specific goal in mind at the outset, such as presenting the findings of a research project. Other times, though, generating the idea for the manuscript or deciding how to develop it is more involved. Every manuscript needs a primary message that is communicated to readers; this message directs how the manuscript is then developed.

Before proceeding, the author should be able to answer these questions: What is the purpose of writing the manuscript? Why is this information important for readers? What difference will it make in clinical practice, teaching, administration, and research? The author should be able to answer these questions clearly and succinctly.

Once the purpose of the manuscript is clearly thought out, the author can record it on an index card and keep the card in view during the writing phase. This helps to stay on target as the writing proceeds. Often, novice writers have enthusiasm about a topic but conceptualize ideas that are too global. As a result, the manuscript may contain extraneous information that distracts from the original intent (Muscari, 1998). Being able to write the purpose of the manuscript in one sentence is a way to assure a clear focus for the article.

Deciding on Importance of Topic

After deciding on the purpose of the manuscript, the author needs to ask if the ideas to be presented are worth writing about. Huth (1999) recommended applying the "so-what test" to the manuscript. This test asks if the message in the manuscript is important enough for publication. The goal in this step in the writing process is to avoid preparing a manuscript that has a limited chance of being accepted for publication.

Display 1.1 presents questions that the author can ask to evaluate if the manuscript is worth writing and if the content is important enough to warrant publication. The author should answer these questions before spending any more time on the manuscript.

Search for Related Articles

In generating ideas for a manuscript, the author should keep in mind that journals are interested in publishing new ideas and communicating new information to readers. If the topic or idea is not new, then the question is whether it presents a new perspective to an existing practice or a different way of looking at a well-known topic.

To determine this, the author should do a literature review on the topic and related content areas. The literature search may reveal that the topic is indeed

DISPLAY 1.1	Assessing Importance of Content of Manuscript

- Does the manuscript present new ideas?
- Is the topic already in the literature? If so, how does the planned manuscript differ from the existing literature?
- If the content is not new and articles already have been published with similar content, what is different about the manuscript to be worthy of publication? What new perspective is offered?
- If the manuscript is published, how important is the message? Will it make a difference in patient care? Will it change nursing practice, education, administration, management, or research?
- Who is the audience, and will readers be interested in the topic?
- Is this a manuscript that a journal would be interested in publishing?

new to the nursing literature or at least to the readers for whom the manuscript is intended. An article may have been published for the general nursing audience, but the intended manuscript focuses instead on how the content would be used by nurses in a specialty area. Or, the articles are research oriented and the intended topic is related to clinical practice or professional issues. If articles have been published on the same topic, they may have been published in journals other than those targeted for the manuscript being planned, or the current focus will add to what is already known about the topic. If the manuscript is not timely and does not present new information, the effort in writing it is wasted (Fondiller, 1999, p. 14).

The goal in searching the literature at this point is to scan articles to determine if others have been published already on the same topic. Do not spend much time with the search in case the decision is made not to write about that topic because it has already been addressed in the literature. If the author finds, though, that the manuscript will present new information, this beginning literature search may be used later as the manuscript is developed. Therefore, record complete information about the articles reviewed for ease in returning to them at a later time.

The next steps in the process of writing for publication are to identify the audience to whom the manuscript will be directed and to select a journal that might be interested in publishing it. These steps are discussed in the next chapter. The goal is to match the topic and type of manuscript with an appropriate journal and readers who would interested in it.

Types of Articles

The topic indicates the type of article to be written. Although articles in the nursing and health care literature can be categorized in many ways, one way is to list them under the following headings: research, clinical practice, professional issue, philosophical and theoretical, review, and other forms of writing such as case reports, book reviews, and writing for consumer and non-professional audiences. These types of manuscripts differ in their goals, format, and often writing style, and frequently they reach different audiences. A manuscript needs to fit the goals of the journal and its readership. Often, manuscripts are rejected because they do not match the type of articles that the journal publishes. Identifying the type of manuscript, therefore, helps the author to make a decision about possible journals for submission (discussed in Chapter 2).

Research Articles

Research articles present the findings of quantitative and qualitative research. Quantitative research papers typically follow the IMRAD format—introduction, methods, results, and discussion—or an adaptation of this, depending on the journal and type of research. There is no one style, however, for presenting qualitative research findings; the format necessarily depends on the purpose of the research, methods, and data (Sandelowski, 1998). With some manuscripts, the intent is to present the original research study, whereas other papers emphasize the clinical implications of the study. Whether the manuscript focuses on original research or the implications of the findings often determines the journals to be considered for submission. The goals of *Nursing Research*, for example, are to report quantitative and qualitative research, present critiques of methodology and research design, and serve as a medium for the stimulation of ideas and exchange of information about nursing research (*Nursing Research*, 2000). Although these articles may discuss clinical and other implications of the research, the focus is more on the research itself. Many clinical practice journals also publish papers on research in their area of practice, and these generally emphasize the clinical implications of the study.

Clinical Articles

A second type of manuscript addresses topics in clinical practice. Clinical articles may be written for nurses across specialties or for nurses practicing in a particular clinical area. The goal of the *American Journal of Nursing* (AJN) is to provide comprehensive and in-depth information to help nurses across different specialties and settings stay current in their profession (*American Journal of Nursing*, 2000). In contrast, articles in journals such as *Cancer Nursing* are more focused on specific patient populations and health problems.

The format for writing clinical articles differs with the journal but usually includes a description of the patient problems and nursing interventions, with an emphasis on the clinical implications of the topic that is presented. Some journals have different departments, each of which has a certain format for its articles.

Professional Issue Articles

Another type of article addresses professional issues. Journals such as the *Online Journal of Issues in Nursing* (OJIN) provide a forum for discussion of pertinent issues in nursing. The intent of this journal is to present different views on topics that affect nursing (*Online Journal of Issues in Nursing*, 2000). Some clinical journals have a department or column on professional issues affecting nurses in that area of clinical practice, societal issues facing patients, and other opinion pieces. Often, the format of these articles depends on the journal, so the author should review the guidelines before writing.

Philosophical and Theoretical Articles

Other topics may be philosophical or may deal with theory development or testing. The format used to develop these manuscripts relates to the goals of the manuscript, philosophical theory used for its development or the position taken, or structure of the theory or framework.

Review Articles

For an integrative review article, the author identifies past research on a particular topic, critiques these studies, and then draws conclusions about the findings. The review of the literature is guided by a research question or problem to be solved. The goal is to identify all of the studies that address the research question. Beyea and Nicoll (1998) differentiated an integrative review article from a literature review and meta-analysis. A literature review is an introduction to new research findings or ideas presented in a manuscript or provides the basis for a proposed study. A meta-analysis extends the critique of the research articles to include statistical analysis of the outcomes of similar studies.

Other Types of Articles

Other forms of writing include case reports, book reviews, and writing for consumer and nonprofessional audiences. Case reports, also termed case studies, provide new information on nursing practice or care of patients with particular health problems by presenting an actual case. The case may be unique or may demonstrate how to plan and deliver care for a patient, family, or community. These manuscripts often begin with why the case was selected and its importance to nursing practice and continue with a description of the patient and related care given by nurses and other disciplines. Nurses also might complete book reviews, describing what the book is about and addressing its quality. Articles might be written for consumers and nonprofessional audiences. The task with this form of writing is to avoid using technical terms and to develop the manuscript at a level that readers without any health care background can understand.

Manuscripts also address topics in nursing education, administration, management, and other nonclinical areas. Articles may be written about research in these areas, or they may describe innovations, new practices, and issues in teaching, administration, and management. Some of these articles describe current practices, whereas others are more philosophical.

Writing Phase

The writing phase involves preparing the first and subsequent drafts of the manuscript, completing the final revision, and submitting the manuscript to the journal. The steps in the writing phase include the following:

1. Develop a formal or an informal outline as a guide to writing.
2. Write the first draft focusing on presenting the content rather than on grammar, spelling, punctuation, and writing style.
3. Revise the first and later drafts continuing to focus on the content of the manuscript.
4. Then revise the manuscript for grammar, spelling, punctuation, and writing style.
5. Prepare tables, figures, and references, paying close attention to the journal's format for references.
6. Prepare the final copy of the manuscript, accompanying materials required by the journal, and the submission letter and send the required copies of the manuscript to the journal's office.

Publishing Phase

The final phase in writing for publication occurs after the manuscript is submitted for publication. The manuscript is critiqued by peer reviewers and the editor, who makes the decision whether to publish it. Editors of nursing journals are professional nurses who have expertise in the content area of the journal. They are peers of the journal's authors and readers who, by their experience and interest, act on their behalf (Fletcher & Fletcher, 1998). Through this process, the best articles are accepted for publication, ensuring quality of information and meeting ethical standards.

Different editorial decisions are possible, ranging from acceptance of the manuscript without revision, a request that the manuscript be revised and resubmitted, and last, to rejection. The publishing phase also includes the responsibilities of the author once the manuscript is accepted for publication.

These steps are as follows:

- Review the critique of the manuscript by the editorial and peer reviewers and revise accordingly.
- If the manuscript is rejected, revise as needed using feedback from the peer review process and submit it to another journal.
- Once accepted for publication, answer queries, carefully read and correct the page proofs, and return all materials to the publisher promptly.

 SUMMARY

Writing for publication is an important skill for nurses to develop. By communicating new initiatives and innovations in clinical practice, findings of research, and other ideas about nursing, nurses direct the future of their practice and advance the development of the profession. There are barriers to writing, but the nurse can overcome these by setting due dates for completion of writing projects, using personal strategies to meet these deadlines, and wisely using the limited time available.

The author begins with an idea, chooses a journal with readers who are interested in that topic, and gears the content and format toward the journal. Selecting a journal is discussed in the next chapter.

Writing for publication is hard work, but the satisfaction gained from completing a manuscript and making a lasting contribution to the literature outweighs the effort and time. Writing is a skill that can be developed with practice. Once a manuscript is completed, the author should begin planning the next one.

REFERENCES

American Association of Colleges of Nursing. (1999) Position statement on nursing research. [On-line]. Available: *http://www.aacn.nche.edu/publications/positions/rscposst.html*. Accessed November 29, 1999.

American Journal of Nursing. (2000). Author guidelines. [On-line]. Available: *http://www.nursingcenter.com/journals*. Accessed March 15, 2000.

Ashworth, P. (1998). Nurses now read more: What about writing too? *Intensive and Critical Care Nursing, 14,* 107.

Beyea, S.C., & Nicoll, L.H. (1998). Writing an integrative review. *AORN Journal, 67,* 877–880.

Bragadóttir, H. (1998). Every nurse can be an author: On writing for publication. *Nursing Forum, 33*(4), 29–32.

Fletcher, R.H., & Fletcher, S.W. (1998). The future of medical journals in the western world. *Lancet, 352*(175), SII30–SII33.

Fondiller, S.H. (1994). Writing for publication. *American Journal of Nursing, 94*(8), 62–65.

Fondiller, S.H. (1999). *The writer's workbook* (2nd ed.). Sudbury, MA: Jones & Bartlett.

Halm, M.A. (1997). Getting published. *American Journal of Nursing, 97*(8), 65–66.

Henninger, D.E., & Nolan, M.T. (1998). A comparative evaluation of two educational strategies to promote publication by nurses. *Journal of Continuing Education in Nursing, 29*, 79–84.

Huth, E.J. (1999). *Writing and publishing in medicine* (3rd ed.). Baltimore: Lippincott Williams & Wilkins.

McConnell, C.R. (1999). From idea to print: Writing for a professional journal. *Health Care Supervisor, 17*(3), 72–85.

Muscari, M.E. (1998). Do the write thing: Writing the clinically focused article. *Journal of Pediatric Health Care, 12*, 236–241.

Nursing Research. (2000). Author guidelines. [On-line]. Available: *http://www.nursingcenter.com/journals/author.cfm*. Accessed March 15, 2000.

Oermann, M.H. (1999a). Extensive writing projects: Tips for completing them on time. *Nurse Author & Editor, 9*(1), 8–10.

Oermann, M.H. (1999b). Writing for publication as an advanced practice nurse. *Nursing Connections, 12*(3), 5–13.

Online Journal of Issues in Nursing. (2000). Information for authors. Available: *http://www.nursingworld.org/ojin/admin/ojinwrtr.html*. Accessed March 18, 2000.

Plawecki, H.M. (1994). Write right! *Journal of Holistic Nursing, 12*, 135–137.

Sandelowski, M. (1998). Writing a good read: Strategies for re-presenting qualitative data. *Research in Nursing and Health, 21*, 375–382.

Sheridan, D.R., & Dowdney, D.L. (1997). *How to write and publish articles in nursing* (2nd ed.). New York: Springer.

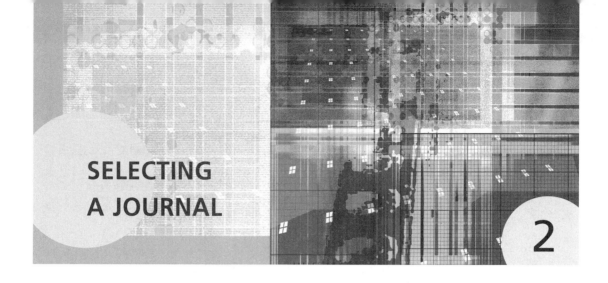

SELECTING A JOURNAL

2

The first step in writing for publication is to identify the topic or focus of the paper. The next steps are to identify the audience to whom the manuscript will be directed and to select a journal that might be interested in publishing it. How to review possible journals, select an appropriate one, and write a query letter are discussed in this chapter.

WHO IS THE AUDIENCE?

The author needs to be clear as to the intended readers of the manuscript. Identifying the audience is an important step because the manuscript needs to be written for defined readers and then submitted to a journal that publishes manuscripts on that topic for the same audience. Otherwise, the manuscript will be inappropriate for the journal to which it has been submitted. A manuscript written for a general nursing audience but then submitted to a specialty journal read predominantly by nurses in advanced practice probably will be rejected, and the author will lose valuable time.

The author can begin by asking who is likely to read the manuscript and benefit by its content. Most articles are read by people who need answers to questions about their practice, teaching, management, or research or about other aspects of their work. Early decisions about the audience include whether the readers are nurses in general practice or in a specialized area of nursing practice; whether they are staff nurses, advanced practice nurses, faculty, managers, or nurses in other roles; whose needs would be met from reading the manuscript; and who would benefit from the content in the manuscript. Display 2.1 provides questions to help the author decide on the audience of the manuscript.

Identifying the Audience of Manuscript

- For whom will the article be written?
- Is the manuscript geared to a specialized audience, or is the content intended for nurses in general?
- If specialized, what is the reader's area of clinical nursing practice (eg, pediatrics)?
- What is the primary role of the reader, such as staff nurse, advanced practice nurse, educator, and manager, which would influence how the manuscript is written?
- What is the work setting (eg, hospital) of the reader?
- Which of the reader's needs will be met by the manuscript?
- How will the information improve the reader's practice, teaching, management, research, or other aspects of work?
- What should the intended reader already know about the content area, and how will the manuscript build on this understanding?
- What is the educational level of the audience?

The audience also may be consumers. Many health journals written for the public may have nurses contributing articles. Writing for patients and consumers influences the depth and complexity of the content, technical words used in the writing, presentation style, and length of the manuscript.

Once the readers of the manuscript are clarified, the author should record this information for use in selecting journals. During the writing process, the author keeps the intended audience in mind when deciding on the content and how it is presented to the readers, types of examples to use, and writing style.

 ## CONSIDERATIONS IN CHOOSING A JOURNAL

Deciding on a journal is an early step in writing for publication. Journals differ widely in their goals, the types of articles published, and writing styles. Selecting an appropriate journal is important because the author's goal is to submit the manuscript to a journal that publishes articles in the subject area that is consistent with the type of manuscript planned (eg, a research report). The choice of journals targeted for submission, therefore, should be carefully made; otherwise, it is unlikely that the manuscript will be accepted.

If a paper is submitted to an inappropriate journal, three actions may occur. First, the editor may return the manuscript to the author without being reviewed. The editor may determine that the paper is unsuitable for the journal. Second, the paper may be reviewed but then rejected because of its lack of fit with the journal's mission and readers. The comments made by reviewers, though, may not facilitate revision because of their lack of expertise in the specialty area. With these first two possibilities, valuable time is lost. Third, the manuscript may be accepted and subsequently published but in a journal never read by nurses who need the information for their practice.

Match With Topic

The primary consideration in selecting a journal is whether the journal publishes articles in the subject area of the proposed manuscript. Is the topic appropriate for the journal? Although the author may be familiar with prominent journals in a particular area of nursing, other journals also may publish articles on the topic or in related content areas. The author should review all possible journals in nursing and other health fields that might be interested in the manuscript and should keep a list of them with related materials such as author guidelines. If an editor is not interested in reviewing the proposed manuscript or the manuscript is rejected, then the author has other possible journals to consider for submission.

Match With Type of Article

The second consideration in choosing a journal is whether it publishes the type of article being planned. Different types of articles were identified in Chapter 1: research, clinical practice, issue, theoretical, review, case reports, and others. The journals appropriate for the topic may not publish the type of manuscript being considered. For instance, the goal of the proposed manuscript may be to present research on teaching effectiveness. Whereas *Nurse Educator* publishes articles on teaching and the role of the teacher, it typically does not publish research reports. The *Journal of Nursing Education*, which publishes research, would be more appropriate. If the intended manuscript will provide a critical review of the literature in a particular area of nursing practice, then the author needs to identify a journal that publishes comprehensive reviews rather than short descriptions of innovations in clinical practice.

The review of journals also guides the author in planning the manuscript. From this review, the author develops ideas on how to write the manuscript to better fit the journal for submission and about other possible directions for the manuscript.

Match With Intended Audience

The third consideration is whether the readers of the journal are the same as the intended audience of the manuscript. Every journal has its own readers and style of presentation that meets their needs. There is a primary audience—readers for whom the journal is targeted—and a secondary audience—people outside of the journal's target audience who read an article to meet a particular need. The goal, however, is to learn as much as possible about the primary or target audience of the journal. The primary audience may be highly specialized and narrow in focus, or the journal may be geared to a general readership. The primary audience for the *Journal of Intravenous Nursing*, for instance, is nurses involved in the administration of intravenous therapy to patients, a specialized area of nursing practice, compared with the *American Journal of Nursing*, whose primary audience is nurses in general. The choice of journals for manuscript submission depends on the targeted audience (Muscari, 1998).

Learning about the readers also is valuable in preparing the manuscript for a particular journal so that its content, format, and writing style are appropriate. The author typically can learn about the readers by reviewing the journal's Information for Authors page (described later) and sample articles in the journal.

In reviewing journals, the author may decide to gear the manuscript toward a different audience to expand the possible journals for submission. The author may have planned to develop a manuscript for critical care nurses but realized from the review that nurses working in noncritical care settings would benefit more from the information, thereby expanding the choice of publications.

Quality of Journal

Three other considerations in selecting a journal include the quality of the journal, its circulation, and how frequently it is published. There is no system for ranking the quality of nursing journals. The author often can judge the quality and prestige of the journals by identifying the ones in which important papers have been published. Reading selected articles in the journals being considered provides an opportunity for the author to evaluate the quality of the articles, whether they present new and important information for readers, and if they are well written—other indicators of the journal's quality.

Another way of assessing the quality of the journal is by reviewing the number of times articles in one journal are cited in other publications. The *Journal Citation Reports®* counts the number of articles published in each journal and the number of times each article has been cited by other scholarly publications, and then calculates an impact factor. The impact factor is the number of current citations to articles published in a specific journal in a 2-year period divided by the total number of articles published in the same journal over the same 2-year period (Institute for Scientific Information, 2000). The *Journal Citation Reports* Science Edition provides citation data on more than 5,700 leading science journals; the Social Sciences Edition provides citation data on approximately 1,700 leading social sciences journals (Institute for Scientific Information, 2000). The *Journal Citation Reports* is useful if intending to publish in medical or social science journals. There are limited nursing journals, though, in the citation database.

Circulation of Journal

Although the quality of the journal is important, the circulation of the journal also may be considered. Manuscripts are time-consuming to prepare, and authors want to reach as many nurses as possible who will be interested in the topic and can use the new information in their practice. The circulation, though, typically is not a major consideration in deciding on journals for submission. In addition, circulation may not equate with quality of the publication.

One way to identify the circulation of a journal is through *Ulrich's International Periodicals Directory* (2000). The Ulrich directory includes the cost of the journal, frequency of publication, publisher and contact information, the editor's name, circulation, indexes, and whether it is refereed. Another way to gauge circulation is through *PubList.com*, an Internet directory of publications (PubList.com, 2001). The author can search this database on journals, newsletters, and other periodicals. Circulation figures are found in the full record of the journal. The record on *Orthopaedic Nursing*, for instance, indicates that it is published bimonthly, is the journal of the National Association of Orthopaedic Nurses, and has a circulation of 10,000.

Frequency of Publication

One final consideration is the frequency with which the journal is published. The time from acceptance to publication of a manuscript usually is less for a monthly journal than a quarterly one (Day, 1998). For journals that publish the acceptance date of the manuscript, the author easily can determine the length of time between acceptance and publication. Remember that many journals, monthly, bimonthly and quarterly, have backlogs; the projected time between acceptance and publication may be a factor in choosing the journals for publication. It is sometimes worthwhile to ask colleagues about their experiences in publishing in a journal and the length of time from submission through publication.

TOOLS FOR IDENTIFYING JOURNALS

To choose the "right" journal for the manuscript, the author needs to review available journals in nursing and other health fields. There are several ways to identify possible journals.

Key Nursing Journals Chart

A valuable resource for reviewing nursing journals is the Key Nursing Journals Chart© (Allen, 2000a). The chart is available as a PDF (portable document format) file or Microsoft Word file at the Nursing and Allied Health Resources Section (NAHRS) of the Medical Library Association Web site at *http://www.library.kent.edu/nahrs/resource/reports/specrpts.html*.

The chart describes characteristics of nursing journals, including the following:

- If they are peer reviewed
- The percentage and number of research articles published in each journal, derived from the Cumulative Index to Nursing and Allied Health Literature® (CINAHL) database searches
- Indexes in which they are listed
- If abstracts and references are available
- Where to obtain full-text articles on line, if available.

The chart is helpful in identifying journals that are peer reviewed and that publish research. Most of the journals in nursing are peer reviewed, even though the review process may differ widely across the journals. The information in the chart is particularly useful if the author is planning to write a research manuscript. For instance, the *Journal of Nursing Scholarship* is peer reviewed and published 90 (44%) research articles in a 2-year period. In contrast, in the *AORN Journal* (by the Association of Operating Room Nurses), which also is peer reviewed, only 30 (6%) of the articles published during the same time period were research reports (Allen, 2000a).

The chart also may be used to identify journals that might be interested in a research report in a specific clinical area. If the manuscript is on research in critical care nursing, for example, the chart may be used to select journals that publish these studies. The *American Journal of Critical Care* had 105 (57%) research articles in a 2-year period, similar to *Heart & Lung* (102 articles, or 56%). *Critical Care Nurse*, in contrast, published only seven (3%) research articles in the same time period (Allen, 2000a). An article that describes a critical care research project would be more suited for submission to the *American Journal of Critical Care* or *Heart & Lung* than to *Critical Care Nurse*. The author then can go to the Web sites, if available, of the prospective journals to review the table of contents of recent issues to confirm their appropriateness. For instance, the Web page of the *American Journal of Critical Care* (2000) provides abstracts of its articles that confirm the extent of research published in the journal.

Another resource to identify journals that publish nursing research is the Top Research Journals Chart, also developed by Allen (2000b). This chart includes nursing journals with 60% or more of their substantive articles on research or that published 72 or more research articles in the years 1996 to 1998.

CINAHL Database

The CINAHL database has been a comprehensive guide to nursing and allied health literature since 1982. There are 1,232 journals currently indexed in

CINAHL, including 417 nursing journals, 281 allied health journals, 413 biomedical journals, and 56 consumer health journals (CINAHL, 2000a). The complete list of journals is available in the print index of CINAHL and on line (CINAHL, 2000b).

CINAHL can be used to review the journals that published articles about the topic of the manuscript and in related content areas. The author can find this information by doing a subject search. This often assists the author in identifying journals that might be interested in the manuscript and in determining if the idea is new or already is in the literature. By reviewing the abstracts of the articles, the author can learn more about the focus of the journal and types of papers published in it.

There also are databases to retrieve material specific to clinical specialties. These databases include a list of journals in each specialty area such as advanced practice nursing, case management, critical care, and emergency care, which the author can use to identify possible journals (CINAHL, 2000c).

Directories of Journals

Some Web sites provide directories of journals in nursing and other health fields (See Display 2.4, p. 26). These sites contain an alphabetical listing of hundreds of journal titles. Many of the sites have links to the Information for Authors page of the journal as well as email addresses of editors for querying them about the proposed manuscript. They do not describe characteristics of the journals, though, as does the Key Nursing Journals Chart, but they provide easy access to editors for the author to direct queries about manuscript ideas.

INFORMATION FOR AUTHORS

After identifying possible journals, the author should read the Information for Authors page—also referred to as Author Guidelines and Instructions for Contributors—from the journals being considered. The Information for Authors page usually describes the following:

- Topics of interest to the journal
- Types of articles published (eg, research, clinical practice, case studies, and commentaries)
- Requirements of manuscript preparation, including the title page, abstract, text, references, figures, tables, photographs, permission to reprint, and copyright transfer
- Editorial process, peer review, and related information
- Length of manuscripts
- Guidelines for submitting the manuscript.

The Information for Authors page may be found in each issue of the journal or in a specific issue, such as the first one of a volume (ie, January). Typically, this page also is available at the Web site of the journal and therefore may be easily obtained once the potential journals have been selected.

For most journals, the author guidelines are consistent with the Uniform Requirements for Manuscripts Submitted to Biomedical Journals (International Committee of Medical Journal Editors, 1997). Sometimes referred to as the "Vancouver Style," the Uniform Requirements are instructions to authors on how to prepare manuscripts.

After reviewing the author guidelines and narrowing the list of possible journals, the author should read a few articles in each journal to get a better perspective on the types of papers published, their format and length, and the writing style. It is helpful to keep a file of author guidelines and sample articles from these journals for use with the current and later writing projects.

 ## MAKING THE DECISION

Display 2.2 provides a check list to help the author decide on the right journal. In making this decision, the author considers the appropriateness of the journal for the topic, type of manuscript, the intended audience, and the quality of the journal. The journals identified for submission, though, may not be the ones with the most important papers, nor the ones cited more frequently by other authors. The journals chosen for the manuscript should be ones read by nurses who are interested in the topic and need the information. Thus, with many manuscripts, the decision as to which journals are appropriate weighs heavily on who reads the journal, who "cares about" the content in the manuscript, and who will use it for improved practice.

One other consideration is the risk of rejection. Prestigious journals also receive more manuscripts for review and have higher rates of rejection. With rejections, the author loses the time that it took for the manuscript to be processed and reviewed. Huth (1999) suggested that sometimes the best choice of a journal may not be the top journal in the field, but another one with a lower risk of rejection that is read by or at least known by the intended audience.

Prioritizing Journals for Submission

From the review of journals, the author should select three to five journals for submission of the manuscript and should prioritize them. If the editor

✔ Does the journal publish articles in the general subject area of the manuscript?
✔ Is the topic of the manuscript consistent with the goals and mission of the journal?
✔ Has the topic of the manuscript been published already in the journal? If so, will the manuscript be different enough to warrant publication?
✔ Does the journal publish the type of manuscript proposed (eg, research, clinical practice, issue, theoretical, review articles, or case reports)?
✔ Who are the readers of the journal, and are they the same as the intended audience of the manuscript?
✔ What is the quality of the journal, and does it publish important articles?
✔ What is the circulation of the journal?
✔ How frequently is the journal published (eg, monthly, bimonthly, quarterly)?
✔ What is the projected time between acceptance and publication?
✔ Is the journal peer reviewed?
✔ Is the journal editor interested in reviewing the manuscript?

of the journal of first choice is not interested in reviewing the manuscript or it is rejected, then the author can send the manuscript to the next one on the list without having to again review the journals.

The author also can prepare a secondary list of journals that publish related topics or may be appropriate if the manuscript is adapted for their audience. This list is valuable if the primary journals are not interested in reviewing the manuscript, the author decides not to submit it to one of them, or the manuscript is rejected. Often, the manuscript can be adapted to another journal without much effort. For instance, if the manuscript is on nursing interventions for dyspnea and the primary journals are not interested in reviewing it, the author might reframe the discussion around caring for the dyspneic patient in the home. Then, the choice of journals extends to those that focus on home care. For rejected manuscripts, the author might refer to this secondary list of publications for ideas about how to rewrite the manuscript to better fit those journals. A research report, for instance, that has been rejected because of a small sample size may be rewritten as a clinical project with greater emphasis placed on the implications of the study.

Query Letter

A query letter can be sent to the editors of the prospective journals asking about their interest in reviewing the manuscript. The author does not need to send a query letter, though, before submitting a manuscript, but it often saves time in the long run. The editor may not be interested in reviewing the manuscript because the journal does not publish that topic or type of manuscript, the journal recently has published too many articles on related topics, or a similar one has already been accepted.

Query letters may be sent to more than one editor simultaneously. The manuscript, however, may be sent to only one journal at a time. After deciding on the journal for manuscript submission, the author should notify the other interested editors of the decision not to send the manuscript for review.

The query letter should be no longer than one page. It should indicate the type of manuscript, for example, description of clinical practice innovation, research report, or case review, and should explain in a few sentences what the manuscript is about. In the query letter, the author should include a tentative title of the manuscript, a brief statement of the author's position and expertise to write the manuscript, the anticipated completion date, and contact information. Black (1995) cautioned authors to avoid trying to "sell" the editor on the topic because the topic should sell itself. A sample query letter is in Display 2.3.

The query letter should be addressed to the editor. This information is available in most of the directories of journals but also may be found at the Web page of the journal, at the publisher's Web site, or in the masthead of a current issue of the journal. Querying editors is done easily by email using the addresses or links available in the directories of journals, such as those in Display 2.4, or at the journal's Web page. The author also may send a letter to the editor. In the latter case, a self-addressed and stamped envelope should be enclosed, or an email address for the response should be given in the letter.

 SUMMARY

The first step in writing for publication is to identify the topic or focus of the manuscript. From that point, the author decides on the intended readers. The manuscript needs to be written for defined readers and then submitted to a journal that publishes articles on that topic for the same audience.

Considerations in selecting a journal include whether the journal publishes articles in the subject area of the proposed manuscript; whether it publishes the type of article being planned (eg, research, clinical practice, issue, theoretical, review, or case report); whether the readers of the journal are the same as the intended audience of the manuscript; the quality of the journal; its circulation; and how frequently it is published.

DISPLAY
2.3 **Sample Query Letter**

Mary Smith, RN, BSN
1224 Moss Street
Reading, PA 19709

January 6, 2002

Marilyn Oermann, PhD, RN, FAAN
Editor, *Outcomes Management*
5557 Cass Avenue
Detroit, MI 48202

Dear Dr. Oermann:

I am interested in submitting a manuscript to *Outcomes Management.* The manuscript describes an evaluation we conducted of a new teaching program for patients with congestive heart failure. For our evaluation, we collected information about the learning needs of patients when they were first admitted to the hospital and assessed the effectiveness of our teaching program at two points in time: at discharge and 1 month after discharge. I have extensive experience caring for patients with cardiac problems and chaired the group that developed and evaluated the teaching program.

The manuscript will be completed by February 2002. Thank you for your consideration.

Sincerely,

Mary Smith, RN, BSN
Clinical Nurse II

There are several ways to identify possible journals. These include the Key Nursing Journals Chart (Allen, 2000a), the CINAHL database, and Web sites that provide directories of nursing and allied health journals. Many of the Web sites have links to the Information for Authors page of the journal and to the editors for querying them about the proposed manuscript.

The author selects three to five journals for submission of the manuscript and prioritizes them. A query letter can be sent to the editors of the prospective journals asking about their interest in reviewing the manuscript. Other decisions made before writing the manuscript are discussed in Chapter 3.

DISPLAY 2.4   Web Sites of Directories of Journals

http://members.aol.com/suzannehj/naed.html

This site is the On-Line Nursing Editors' Page, which provides an index of editors of nursing journals and books with e-mail connections. When publishers have author guidelines on a Web site, these direct URL sites also are included. More than 140 journals are listed alphabetically, as well as 8 book editors.

http://www.son.utmb.edu/catalog/catalog.html

The Academic Journal Directory of the University of Texas Medical Branch School of Nursing at Galveston contains listings for more than 400 professional academic journals in clinical nursing, nursing education, nursing research, and related health care fields. A typical entry contains the full name of the journal, its publisher, its frequency of publication, its intended readership, the types of manuscripts reviewed, and a statement of purpose for prospective authors. The contact address for each journal is included with links to most journals' and publishers' Web sites.

http://www.nursingcenter.com

NursingCenter.com includes a list of journals with the table of contents of current and past issues, information about the journal, author guidelines, and links to the editors. Authors can print the author guidelines and other information about the journal and e-mail the editors directly from this Web site. In addition, NursingCenter.com provides full-text nursing journal articles.

http://www.mco.edu/lib/instr/libinsta.html

This list contains links to Web sites that provide instructions to authors for more than 3,000 journals in the health and life sciences. All links are to "primary sources," that is, to publishers or organizations with editorial responsibilities for the journals. The journals are listed alphabetically.

http://www.lib.umich.edu/hw/nursing/resources.html

This site includes journals with full-text articles on-line and free of charge, author information pages for many journals, and access to other nursing resources. The journals are listed alphabetically with links to the Web site of the journal.

http://www.library.kent.edu/nahrs/resource/reports/specrpts.html

The Web site for the Nursing and Allied Health Resources Section (NAHRS) of the Medical Library Association provides access to the Key Nursing Journals Chart© developed by Allen (2000a). The chart is available in two formats: a PDF file or Microsoft Word file. The Key Nursing Journals Chart describes characteristics of nursing journals including if they are peer reviewed, the percentage and number of research articles published in each journal, indexes in which they are listed, if abstracts and references are available, and where to obtain full-text articles, if available.

REFERENCES

Allen, M. (2000a). Key nursing journals: Characteristics and database coverage, 2000 ed. [On-line]. Available: *http://www.library.kent.edu/nahrs/resource/reports/specrpts.html*. Accessed December 15, 2000.

Allen, M. (2000b, January). Nursing journals: No, they're not all online for free. *Nursing and Allied Health Resources Section Newsletter, 20*(1), 7–9.

American Journal of Critical Care (2000). [On-line]. Available: *http://www.aacn.org*. Accessed April 29, 2000.

Black, J. (1995). Writing for publication: Advice to potential authors. *Plastic Surgical Nursing, 16*, 90–93.

CINAHL. (2000a). The CINAHL database. [On-line]. Available: *http://www.cinahl.com/prodsvcs/cinahldb.html*. Accessed May 2, 2000.

CINAHL. (2000b). List of journal titles currently indexed in the CINAHL database. [On-line]. Available: *http://www.cinahl.com/library/jour000412.PDF*. Accessed May 2, 2000.

CINAHL. (2000c). Update on the CINAHL database and what's new for 1999: Special interest categories. [On-line]. Available: *http://www.cinahl.com/prodsvcs/dbupdate1999.html*. Accessed May 2, 2000.

Day, R.A. (1998). *How to write and publish a scientific paper* (5th ed.). Phoenix, AZ: Oryx Press.

Huth, E.J. (1999). *Writing and publishing in medicine* (3rd ed.). Baltimore: Lippincott Williams & Wilkins.

Institute for Scientific Information. (2000). Journal citation reports. [On-line]. Available: *http://www.isinet.com/products/citation/jcr.html*. Accessed April 23, 2000.

International Committee of Medical Journal Editors. (1997). Uniform requirements for manuscripts submitted to biomedical journals. *Annals of Internal Medicine, 126*(1), 36–47. Also available: *http://www.thelancet.com/newlancet/sub/author/uniform1.html*.

McConnell, C.R. (1999). From idea to print: Writing for a professional journal. *Health Care Supervisor, 17*(3), 72–85.

Muscari, M.E. (1998). Do the write thing: Writing the clinically focused article. *Journal of Pediatric Health Care, 12*, 236–241.

PubList.com. (2001). The Internet directory of publications. [On-line serial]. Available: *http://www.publist.com*. Accessed May 2, 2000.

Ulrich's international periodicals directory (39th ed.). (2001). New Providence, NJ: R.R. Bowker.

AUTHORSHIP
AND
PREPARING
TO WRITE

3

Decisions about the focus of the manuscript, audience, and journal are important early in the writing process. Other decisions pertain to authorship; if these are not made before beginning the writing project, they may later create problems and conflict among the authors. This chapter addresses authorship and author responsibilities in preparing to write.

AUTHORSHIP

Each individual designated as an author on a manuscript should have contributed sufficiently to it. Authorship is more than preparing the manuscript; it requires participating in and understanding the research and other types of projects and conveys public responsibility for the work (Gaeta, 1999). The Uniform Requirements for Manuscripts Submitted to Biomedical Journals (International Committee of Medical Journal Editors [ICMJE], 1997) specifies that authorship credit should be given only when the author made substantial contributions to:

1. The conception and design of the study, or to the analysis and interpretation of the data
2. Drafting the manuscript or revising it for important content
3. Approval of the final version of the manuscript.

All three criteria must be met for a person to be designated as an author on a manuscript.

These criteria have important implications for authors. First, each co-author must have participated in the project and generated at least part of the content of the paper. Their participation may have involved identifying the questions for the study and designing it, identifying the need for a clinical project and planning its development, or critiquing and synthesizing the literature. A suggestion to design a study or begin a project does not justify authorship.

Individuals who make important contributions to the analysis and interpretation of the data, even though they may not have been involved in the conception and design of the study, qualify for authorship if they meet the other criteria (ICMJE, 1997; Lundberg & Glass, 1996). Collecting the data for a study or project, however, does not qualify for authorship. The author must have analyzed and interpreted the data leading to the conclusions of the study. For clinical projects involving patients, physicians and nurses who care for patients enrolled in a study do not qualify for authorship unless these three criteria have been met.

Next, authors must participate in writing the paper, critiquing it as a basis for subsequent revisions, or substantially revising the paper. Individuals providing editorial assistance do not qualify for authorship. When writing in groups, Huth (1999) suggested that records be maintained of co-authors' recommendations for revisions of drafts and the outcomes of those suggestions. Authors should be able to document their participation in a group writing activity using logs, data entry sheets, records of meetings held, and drafts of manuscripts (Duncan, 1999). This record-keeping may be important after the paper is published if there are questions about its content or methods.

Last, co-authors take responsibility for the content of the manuscript. All authors of a paper should be able to defend it publicly (Huth, 1999).

Other participants in the project who do not meet the criteria for authorship may be recognized in the acknowledgments (discussed later). Individuals who collected the data, provided statistical support, gave technical support for the project, and contributed in other ways are acknowledged for their assistance rather than cited as co-authors.

First Author

Typically, the first or lead author contributes the most to the project and manuscript. The first author often is the person who initiated and developed the clinical project or, in the case of research, is the primary investigator and is responsible for moving the group toward completion of a manuscript to describe its work. However, this is not always true, and the order of author names may be assigned in different ways.

The first author has more responsibilities associated with writing the paper than do the other authors and may be the most experienced in writing for publication. The first author coordinates preparation of the manuscript.

Whereas the group should determine the roles and responsibilities of each author, some common activities completed by the first author are presented in Display 3.1.

Corresponding Author

The corresponding author communicates with the editor, beginning with the query letter, and is designated as such on the title page of the manuscript or in the cover letter. Although the first author usually is the corresponding author, the group may decide that another person should assume this role.

The corresponding author is the contact between the authors and the editor, discussing revisions to be made, working with the editor to assure that these are adequately made, and returning the revisions and related materials

---

DISPLAY 3.1   Responsibilities of First Author

- ✔ Leads the discussion about authorship; the manuscripts to be prepared, their content, and how to organize each one; the order of author names; who will assume responsibility for different parts of the manuscript and for multiple papers if more than one will be prepared; and the time frame
- ✔ Obtains author guidelines and assures that they are met
- ✔ Arranges for word processing of manuscript
- ✔ Completes own writing assignment
- ✔ Edits drafts and suggests revisions to co-authors
- ✔ Maintains copies of all drafts with dates and notes about revisions
- ✔ Edits a final version of the manuscript for a consistent writing style throughout
- ✔ Reads and corrects the final typed manuscript
- ✔ Facilitates approval of the final manuscript by co-authors, asks each author to date and initial the final copy, indicating their approval of it, and files these
- ✔ Keeps copies of references used in preparing the manuscript and for background work
- ✔ Sets up group meetings and keeps records of the discussions
- ✔ Assures that co-authors adhere to the time frame and takes the actions established by the group when co-authors do not
- ✔ Obtains permissions if needed
- ✔ Makes sure that the correct number of copies of the manuscript and other required materials are submitted with it
- ✔ May assume responsibilities of corresponding author
- ✔ Coordinates subsequent revisions of the manuscript after peer review
- ✔ Coordinates signing of the copyright agreement by co-authors
- ✔ Reviews page proofs, which are the typeset manuscript pages reviewed for errors before publication, and returns them promptly to the publisher

on time. The contact between the corresponding author and editor helps to establish the credibility of the group and its dependability. Positive working relationships between authors and editors are important in terms of future publications. Once the paper is published, the corresponding author communicates with readers by distributing reprints of the article and answering questions.

Co-Authors

Multiple authorship of articles has become the norm (Gaeta, 1999). When writing with multiple authors, the first step is to decide on authorship and who qualifies. Each author must meet the criteria for authorship described earlier in the chapter.

Co-authors assume responsibility not only for their sections of the manuscript, but for the intellectual content of the paper as a whole. All authors of a manuscript need to approve the final version, not only by signing the copyright transfer form, but also by approving the content.

In writing the manuscript, the group should decide on the roles and responsibilities of the co-authors, keeping in mind the criteria for justifying authorship on a paper. Remember that each author should be able to defend the manuscript publicly.

Order of Author Names

The second step when writing with multiple authors is to determine the order of author names. This should be decided at the outset to avoid conflict and problems later on.

The order of co-authors' names should be determined by their relative contributions to the work (Riesenberg & Lundberg, 1990). In a study of 184 Canadian nurses' views on assignment of publication credit, subjects agreed that credit should be based entirely on contribution and not status, and decisions on authorship should be made early to avoid issues later (Butler & Ginn, 1998). Duncan (1999) recommended that the order be put in writing.

Even with specific criteria for authorship specified by the ICMJE (1997), disputes of authorship have increased recently, along with the number of authors listed with papers. Wilcox (1998) reported a significant increase in authorship disputes and recommended enforcement of published authorship standards.

With the growing number of authors listed with publications, it is more difficult to determine the contributions of each person to the project based on the order of author names. Yank and Rennie (1999) analyzed the descriptions by researchers of their contributions to a project to determine how the order of author names listed in the byline of the article corresponded to these contributions. Although the order of author names did not specify the contributions to the project, the first-author position corresponded to a significantly greater number of contributions. It was not clear, however, how co-authors names were listed on the byline and if their order reflected the extent of their contributions. Other studies also have found variability in the contributions of nonfirst authors on a manuscript (Shapiro, Wenger, & Shapiro, 1994).

Yank and Rennie (1999) proposed a new system for acknowledging contributions to a manuscript that (1) recognizes contributors who performed important work that resulted in the article, (2) lists their contributions for readers, (3) lists in the byline only the names of authors who contributed the most to the work, and (4) identifies the authors who take responsibility for the integrity of the work. They recommended that researchers list their contributions to the manuscript and that editors publish them for readers. This provides disclosure of the contributions made to the research and to the manuscript so the contributors can accept credit and responsibility (Rennie, Yank, & Emanuel, 1997). Smith (1997) cautioned that a system such as this must identify the authors who assume ultimate responsibility for the study. An example of a contributor list using this system is found in Display 3.2.

Acknowledgments

Acknowledgments generally are used to recognize people who contributed to the research, the project itself, or preparation of the manuscript but who do not qualify for authorship. In the acknowledgment section of a manuscript, the author can give credit to people who assisted with the work, such as individuals who:

DISPLAY 3.2 **Example of Contributor List**

ARTICLE CITATION

Oermann, M.H., & Templin, T. (2000). Important attributes of quality health care: Consumer perspectives. *Journal of Nursing Scholarship, 32,* 167–172.

NAMES ON BYLINE

Marilyn Oermann and Thomas Templin

CONTRIBUTOR LIST

Marilyn Oermann was the investigator responsible for the design and conduct of the study and for writing the manuscript. Thomas Templin did the statistical analysis and interpretation. Joette Lambert, Christine Weglarz, and Sue Dillon collected the data, and Clare Harris and Jennifer Dammeyer assisted with data interpretation. (Notice that the latter names are not listed in the article citation.)

- Critically reviewed the research proposal, design, or methods
- Gave advice on the project
- Collected the data
- Analyzed the data
- Provided statistical support
- Provided technical support
- Assisted in writing and preparing the manuscript
- Critically reviewed the manuscript.

Acknowledgments also should specify the financial and material support provided for the project (ICMJE, 1997). An example of an acknowledgment for grant support is, "Supported by Heart and Stroke Foundation of Ontario Grant B-2361." (O'Farrell, Murray, & Hotz, 2000).

People who are mentioned in the acknowledgment section of a manuscript must grant permission to include their names. The inclusion of names in the acknowledgment may suggest endorsement of the content of the manuscript; therefore, they should have the opportunity to read the manuscript and consent to be acknowledged.

Honorary and Ghost Authorship

Authorship establishes both the credit and responsibility for work in nursing, other health fields, and science in general. Misuse of authorship undermines this recognition and responsibility. The criteria established by the ICMJE provide a framework for determining who should be included as an author of a manuscript and who does not deserve authorship.

Flanagin and colleagues (1998) conducted a study of honorary and ghost authorship in peer-reviewed medical journals. Honorary authors are people named as authors who do not fit the criteria, such as the department chairperson, faculty advisor of a research project, or nurse manager of the unit where the author works. Ghost authorship is failure to include authors who made significant contributions to the project. Ghost authors may be the actual writers, such as editors and researchers who write the article but are not cited as authors (Rennie & Flanagin, 1994).

Of 809 articles sampled, 19% (n = 156) had evidence of honorary authors, 11% (n = 93) had evidence of ghost authors, and 2% (n = 13) had both (Flanagin et al., 1998). Honorary authorship was found more frequently with review articles and editorials rather than research articles. Awarding authorship to people who did not contribute substantially to the project and manuscript (honorary authors) and not including people who did (ghost authors) suggests a misuse of authorship criteria or a lack of understanding as to who deserves authorship on an article.

MULTIPLE AUTHORS: WORKING TOGETHER

The group involved in writing the manuscript should meet with all members present to discuss these areas: (1) who meets the criteria for authorship and who should be acknowledged instead, (2) the types of manuscripts that might be prepared, (3) the roles and responsibilities of each group member and order of names, and (4) the time frame for completion of the manuscript. As in any group effort, the more co-authors involved in planning and writing the manuscript, the more difficult it is to coordinate the writing efforts and keep track of the group's progress. Each group working on a manuscript should be coordinated by one person who can track progress and keep the group on schedule.

The first responsibility of the group is to review the criteria for authorship and decide who meets them. Other contributors then would be recognized in the acknowledgment. The group may invite a facilitator, who understands the publication process and is not involved in the project, to assist in reaching decisions about authorship and the order of names (Duncan, 1999). Discussions of the group and decisions reached should be recorded by one of the group members and kept in case questions and issues arise later.

The second responsibility of the group is to determine how many and what types of manuscripts will be prepared, including the audiences to be reached and potential journals. If the project involves research, the authors need to decide on how the study findings will be disseminated and whether multiple papers may result and for which types of audiences and journals. If multiple manuscripts may emerge from the work completed by the group, this should be decided in the beginning so the roles and responsibilities associated with preparing the manuscripts may be rotated among the group. Authorship roles may be changed with each manuscript (Duncan, 1999).

The first priority for dissemination of the work is professional journals, but manuscripts also may be prepared for consumer audiences and other non-professional groups. The discussions also might include presentations to be made at conferences, including oral presentations and posters, so that these activities are reflected when the work is divided among the group.

Once the decisions are made about the types and number of manuscripts, the third function of the group is to determine the roles and responsibilities of group members and order of names on each manuscript. The roles and responsibilities may shift as the writing project progresses, and with this shift may come a change in the order of author names. With some manuscripts, there is a natural break in the content, such as the description of a clinical innovation and its evaluation, that may lend itself to dividing the writing among group members (Barnum, 1995). Figure 3-1 is a tracking form for use in group writing projects.

The fourth decision involves establishing a time frame for completion of each phase in the writing project and manuscript as a whole. The time frame

Name of research study, clinical project, manuscript:				
Authors (list in order):				
Acknowledgments (list in order):				
Manuscript responsibilities (list and describe)	**Author assigned**	**Due date**	**Submit to**	**Date completed**

Figure 3-1. Tracking form for group writing projects.

should include the expectations of each group member with accompanying due dates and dates for the group to meet. The discussion of the time frame also should include the actions to be taken if co-authors do not complete their responsibilities by the due date. This is an important area of discussion because if due dates are not established and met, the writing project may never be completed. The actions to be taken when co-authors do not complete their responsibilities on time might include being dropped entirely from the writing group and listed as a contributor in the acknowledgments or involve a change in responsibilities and reordering of author names. Whatever actions are decided by the group should be specified at this point in the discussions rather than when required because of noncompliance. With a written contract the group can specify the expectations of each co-author and consequences of not meeting them (Duncan, 1999).

 FORMAT OF MANUSCRIPT

In this book, the term "paper" is used interchangeably with "manuscript." The unpublished document is the paper or manuscript (American Medical Association, 1998). A paper is submitted to a journal in the form of a manuscript, which eventually may be published or may exist only in the form of a manuscript. When published, the manuscript is referred to as an article.

Before beginning to write, the author should have a clear understanding of the format of the manuscript—the different sections from first to last. "Format" here does not refer to each content area of the manuscript, planned later in the writing project, but instead reflects its general organization. Understanding the format gives the author a sense of where to begin and where to end.

Although there are differences in the types of articles published by journals, manuscripts are organized using a general format beginning with the title page and ending with the figures (illustrations). Differences exist in how the text is structured, depending on whether it is a report of original research, case study, description of clinical practice, or review article, but in general manuscripts are organized in the following order. This is the same order in which the manuscript should be submitted to the journal unless stated otherwise in the author guidelines.

1. Title page
2. Abstract page
3. Text
4. Acknowledgments
5. References
6. Tables
7. Figures.

Each of these sections begins on a new page using double spacing throughout. Pages are numbered consecutively, beginning with the title page, in the upper or lower right-hand corner of each page (ICMJE, 1997) or as indicated by the author guidelines of the journal. Papers of all types should be printed on one side only.

 ## ASSEMBLING MATERIALS FOR WRITING

The author completes other preparations before beginning to write. These preparations include obtaining the author guidelines for the journal; gathering materials about the project, innovation, or practices described in the manuscript; assembling analyses of data and other information about the research project; and deciding on word processing. These preliminary activities are important to allow authors to focus on their writing once they begin rather than focusing on time-consuming and sometimes distracting tasks, such as finding evidence needed to support ideas, locating statistical analyses of data, and checking references.

Information for Authors

The importance of identifying possible journals before beginning to write and obtaining the author guidelines are discussed in Chapter 2. In preparing to write, the author should read these guidelines carefully because they indicate how the manuscript should be developed for different departments in the journal, the page limits for the text, the number of tables and figures allowed, and the reference format. For example, manuscripts may be prepared for four categories in *Nursing Research*: regular articles that are original research reports (limited to 14–16 pages), brief reports of cutting-edge ideas and pilot studies with important results (limited to 8 pages), methodology articles on innovative aspects of the research process (limited to 8 pages), and letters to the editor (less than 450 words) (*Nursing Research*, 2000). The organization of the manuscript, requirements of each section, instructions for typing the paper, and how to save it as an electronic file also are specified in the author guidelines.

Similarly, the information for authors for *Western Journal of Nursing Research* (WJNR) specifies: (1) how research reports should be organized; (2) requirements of each section of the manuscript (ie, the introduction is limited to one paragraph); (3) a page limit of 20 pages maximum, including tables and figures; (4) a limit of three tables and figures; and (5) how to type and submit the paper (*WJNR*, 2000).

The same is true for clinical practice and other types of journals in nursing. The author guidelines for *MCN, The American Journal of Maternal/Child Nursing* (*MCN*), for instance, describe general manuscript preparation and specific instructions for the title, second, third, and fourth pages; references;

and tables and figures (limited to five) (MCN, 2000). The maximum number of pages is 20 including references, tables, and figures. Manuscripts dealing with clinical practice and practice issues begin with an introduction and end with clinical implications. The guidelines emphasize that research papers are considered only if they have strong implications for clinical practice.

The *American Journal of Critical Care* (American Association of Critical-Care Nurses, 2000) publishes multiple types of manuscripts, each with its own word limit. The following types are included:

- Clinical studies (1500–4000 words)
- Basic research studies (1500–4000 words)
- Preliminary/short communications (500–1500 words)
- Case reports (500–1500 words)
- Clinical/basic science reviews, including historical material (1500–4000 words).

These few examples illustrate the importance of having the author guidelines available before writing the manuscript to avoid extensive revisions later. It is easier to plan on writing a 15-page manuscript than to write a 25-page one that needs to be shortened before submission, and to organize the sections of a manuscript so that they are consistent with the journal guidelines rather than reorganize the final version to meet those requirements. Submitting a paper that does not conform to the journal guidelines may result in delays after it is reviewed.

Some journals even restrict the number of references allowed with the manuscript. For example, *MCN* (2000) requests no more than 30 references be included.

If the guidelines do not specify page and table limits, the author might review articles published in the journals being considered to get a sense of their usual length. One journal page represents about three typed and double-spaced manuscript pages; often, no more than three tables and figures are allowed. Knowing the maximum number of tables and figures allowed is important to avoid having to delete some and rewrite the information back into text once the manuscript has already been written.

The author also can contact the editor with questions about specifications of manuscripts or can refer to the Uniform Requirements for Manuscripts Submitted to Biomedical Journals available at *http://www.icmje.org/*.

Related Documents

Before beginning to write, the author should gather documents that might be needed in preparing the manuscript. Most papers are based on background work completed by the author or others and on bibliographic information. The author should assemble documents of this sort before writing to avoid having to locate these materials later and relying on memory. The goal is to have the materials available to facilitate writing the manuscript.

For research papers, the author should assemble these materials at minimum before beginning to write:

- Descriptions of the research project, such as the research proposal; grant applications; and papers on the background of the study, design, methods, and instruments
- Descriptions of the intervention evaluated, which may include illustrations, if relevant
- Results of the literature review completed as background of the study to better understand the findings and to prepare the study for publication
- Findings of the study, including the data analysis, statistical analyses (if relevant), and preliminary tables and figures developed in analyzing the data
- Papers and posters developed by the author for presentation of the research at conferences.

For papers that are not data based, such as manuscripts on projects, innovations, nursing care of patients, and trends in nursing, the author should assemble these materials at minimum before beginning to write:

- Descriptions of the project, innovation, protocol, and nursing care, including illustrations if relevant
- Descriptions of the need for change in nursing practice, education, administration, and other areas of nursing
- Any data analyses from evaluations
- Permissions to use reports from the setting on the background of the project, why a change was needed, and descriptions of the project itself, and permissions to reprint other types of documents in the manuscript
- Information about the specific type of paper to be written and its requirements, such as with case reports, editorials, and book reviews.

WORD PROCESSING

Someone needs to type the paper. With word processing, the preparation of manuscripts and ability to revise drafts have become easier. Authors may chose to type their own papers including drafts and the final version, so that they may revise when needed and at a convenient time. Sheridan and Dowdney (1997) recommended that authors learn to use word processing to speed the editing process, update manuscripts quickly, and always have clean print-outs to edit. If contracting with someone else for word processing, be sure to provide specific instructions on the requirements of the paper, for instance, margins, use of running heads (a short title that identifies the manuscript), placement of headings and subheadings, and pagination, to avoid having to revise these later.

Writing for publication is not a good time to learn a new word processing program. Before beginning to type the manuscript, the author should learn how to set up the pages to meet the journal requirements, include dates to indicate revisions of drafts, use running heads if required, insert page numbers, include symbols to represent statistics and significance levels, and prepare tables.

A procedure should be established for dating the drafts of the paper and when writing as a group, labeling sections written and revised by different authors. This is important to help keep track of contributions and to know whom to contact if there is a question about the substantive content or why a particular revision was made. Some word processing programs have an option to automatically include the date with each draft.

Another feature that is helpful with group writing is line numbering, in which each line of the manuscript is given a number automatically. This makes it easier to revise the manuscript and respond to comments about its content. Using the annotations feature of word processing software helps co-authors communicate comments about specific parts of the manuscript. Knowing how to use the word processing software to mark revisions while editing a paper also is helpful. None of these techniques, though, should be practiced while writing the manuscript but should be mastered before beginning.

 SUMMARY

Each individual designated as an author on a manuscript or other type of paper should have contributed sufficiently to it. The Uniform Requirements for Manuscripts Submitted to Biomedical Journals specify that authorship credit should be given only when the author made substantial contributions to (1) the conception and design of the study, or to the analysis and interpretation of the data; (2) drafting the manuscript or revising it for important content; and (3) the approval of the final version of the manuscript (ICMJE, :997).

Acknowledgments generally are used to recognize people who contributed to the research, project, or preparation of the manuscript but who do not qualify for authorship. People mentioned in the acknowledgment section of a manuscript must grant permission to include their names.

When writing with multiple authors, the first step is to decide on authorship and who qualifies. The second step is to determine the order of author names. Typically the first author contributes the most to the project and manuscript. The order of co-authors' names should be determined by their relative contributions to the work. Co-authors assume responsibility not only for their sections of the manuscript, but for the intellectual content of the paper as a whole.

Authors complete other preparations before beginning to write. These preparations allow authors to focus on their writing once they begin.

REFERENCES

American Association of Critical-Care Nurses. (2000). *American Journal of Critical Care Author Guidelines*. [On-line]. Available: *http://www.aacn.org*. Accessed June 1, 2000.

American Medical Association. (1998). *Manual of style: A guide for authors and editors* (9th ed.). Baltimore: Lippincott Williams & Wilkins.

Barnum, B.S. (1995). *Writing and getting published: A primer for nurses*. New York: Springer.

Butler, L., & Ginn, D. (1998). Canadian nurses' views on assignment of publication credit for scholarly and scientific work. *Canadian Journal of Nursing Research, 30,* 171–183.

Duncan, A.M. (1999). Authorship, dissemination of research findings, and related matters. *Applied Nursing Research, 12,* 101–106.

Flanagin, A., Carey, L.A., Fontanarosa, P.B., Phillips, S.G., Pace, B.P., Lundberg, G.D., & Rennie, D. (1998). Prevalence of articles with honorary authors and ghost authors in peer-reviewed medical journals. *Journal of the American Medical Association, 280,* 222–224.

Gaeta, T.J. (1999). Authorship: "Law" and order. *Academic Emergency Medicine, 6,* 297–301.

Huth, E.J. (1999). *Writing and publishing in medicine* (3rd ed.). Baltimore: Lippincott Williams & Wilkins.

International Committee of Medical Journal Editors. (1997). Uniform requirements for manuscripts submitted to biomedical journals. *Annals of Internal Medicine, 126*(1), 36–47. Also available: *http://www.icmje.org/*.

Lundberg, G.D., & Glass, R.M. (1996). What does authorship mean in a peer-revised medical journal? *Journal of the American Medical Association, 276,* 75.

MCN American Journal of Maternal/Child Nursing. (2000). Author guidelines. *MCN American Journal of Maternal/Child Nursing, 25,* 114.

Nursing Research. (2000). Author guidelines. [On-line]. Available: *http://www.nursingcenter.com/journals*. Accessed May 31, 2000.

O'Farrell, P., Murray, J., & Hotz, S.B. (2000). Psychologic distress among spouses of patients undergoing cardiac rehabilitation. *Heart and Lung, 29,* 97–104.

Pearsall, T.E. (1997). *The elements of technical writing*. Boston: Allyn and Bacon.

Rennie, D., & Flanagin, A. (1994). Authorship! Authorship! Guests, ghosts, grafters, and the two-sided coin. *Journal of the American Medical Association, 271,* 469–471.

Rennie, D., Yank, V., & Emanuel, L. (1997). When authorship fails: A proposal to make contributors accountable. *Journal of the American Medical Association, 278,* 579–585.

Riesenberg, D., & Lindberg, G.D. (1990). The order of authorship: Who's on first? *Journal of the American Medical Association, 264,* 1857.

Shapiro, D.W., Wenger, N.S., & Shapiro, M.F. (1994). The contributions of authors to multiauthored biomedical research papers. *Journal of the American Medical Association, 271,* 438–442.

Sheridan, D.R., & Dowdney, D.L. (1997). *How to write and publish articles in nursing* (2nd ed.). New York: Springer.

Smith, R. (1997). Authorship: Time for a paradigm shift? *British Medical Journal, 314,* 992.

Western Journal of Nursing Research. (2000). Manuscript specifications for the *Western Journal of Nursing Research*. [On-line]. Available: *http://www.ualberta.ca/fonjrnls/Wjnrins.html*. Accessed May 31, 2000.

Wilcox, L.J. (1998). Authorship: The coin of the realm, the source of complaints. *Journal of the American Medical Association, 280,* 216–217.

Yank, V., & Rennie, D. (1999). Disclosure of researcher contributions: A study of original research articles in *The Lancet. Annals of Internal Medicine, 130,* 661–670.

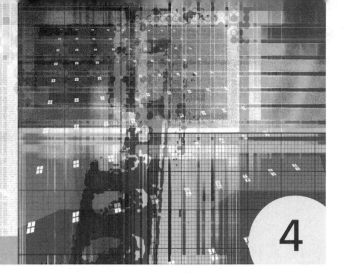

ETHICAL AND LEGAL ISSUES IN WRITING FOR PUBLICATION

4

During the process of writing for publication, authors make many decisions that have important ethical and legal implications (Blancett, 1991). Although the writer often is guided by an editor or publisher in resolving some of these issues, ultimately it is the responsibility of the author to disseminate the work in a manner that maintains scholarly integrity within a profession (Clark, 1993; Cormach, 1991). Ethical and legal issues affecting writing for publication include justified and unjustified authorship; copyright; wasteful or duplicate publication; the submission of fraudulent, false, or fabricated data; plagiarism or misappropriation of the ideas of others; conflict of interest or competing interests among authors and peer reviewers; and privacy rights. This chapter provides an overview of these issues and offers suggestions for preventing or minimizing ethical and legal problems related to writing for publication.

ABUSES OF AUTHORSHIP

Ethical issues related to authorship center around the question of who is entitled to be listed as the author of a scientific publication. Abuses of authorship have been identified as unjustified, irresponsible, and incomplete authorship (Huth, 1986).

Various sources have identified the trend of increasing numbers of articles with multiple authors published in all scientific fields, including health care (Blancett, 1991; Gaeta, 1999; Huth, 1986). Multiple authorship can reflect the increasing complexity of a field, but listing many author names on a short paper suggests that the names of some individuals who were undeserving of authorship have been included (Gaeta, 1999). However, as Huth (1986) pointed out, "Unjustified authorship is not simply a problem of numbers" (p. 257). The central issue may be what Garfield (1995) referred to as "author inflation": giving authorship credit to individuals who made only trivial contributions to published manuscripts.

Authors should understand the standards for authorship qualification developed by the International Committee of Medical Journal Editors (ICMJE, 1997). This set of standards, the Uniform Requirements for Manuscripts Submitted to Biomedical Journals, is used by most medical journals and an increasing number of journals in nursing and other health care disciplines to guide authors in the preparation of manuscripts and to guide editors in confirming appropriate authorship designation.

Issues With Honorary and Ghost Authors

Authorship cannot be conferred on someone as a gift or seized by someone in a position of power; it is a status that can be assumed only voluntarily by an individual who accepts all responsibilities inherent in it (American Medical Association [AMA], 1998, p. 89; Duncan, 1999; Rennie & Flanagin, 1994). The issue is one of gratuitous authorship, which Gaeta (1999) reported to be a prevalent and serious problem among papers published in major scientific journals. It is intellectually dishonest to list as a "guest," "honorary," or "courtesy" author the name of someone who does not meet all criteria for authorship, and it is unlikely that such individuals would be willing or able to take public responsibility for the accuracy of a paper's content if it is challenged. Likewise, it is unethical for a person who is in a position of power over another to claim authorship for self or another (Duncan, 1999).

A related issue is that of "ghost" authorship. In some fields, it is a common practice for a medical writer to be hired to write the manuscript, but this ghost author does not receive authorship credit. Instead, the name of a prominent scientist in that field is attached before the manuscript is submitted. In such cases, neither the person whose name is listed as author nor the ghost writer qualifies for authorship credit, the former because he or she understands the science but is not accountable for the writing, and the latter because she or he can defend the writing but not the science. Ghost authors may be freelance writers who are bound by contract not to receive authorship credit, corporate or governmental agency public relations officers, or authors' editors hired to draft or substantially revise a manuscript (Rennie & Flanagin, 1994). Although they do not qualify as authors, ghost writers should be identified and their contributions explained in an acknowledgment.

Faculty and Student: Authorship Issues

The special case of faculty members and students who author manuscripts may demonstrate elements of guest authorship, ghost authorship, or both. The relative contributions of each person, professor and student, often are perplexing when the student earns academic credit for working on a project and the professor is being compensated for teaching the student. Opinions vary about whether a faculty member who provides guidance to a student, as a normal and expected responsibility of teaching, makes a substantive contribution to that student's manuscript (Butler & Ginn, 1998; Clark, 1993).

Unfortunately, under pressure to publish to meet criteria for tenure and promotion, some faculty members request or demand authorship credit on any manuscript related to student work guided by faculty. However, unless professors meet all three criteria for authorship specified by the Uniform Requirements (ICMJE, 1997), they should not be listed as authors (guest authorship). If a student and a faculty member jointly plan and carry out a project and both contribute to drafting and revising the manuscript, both should be listed as authors. It is unethical for a professor to ask a student to draft a manuscript and not give the student authorship credit, or worse, to assign a paper as a course requirement and then to submit the student's work for publication without listing the student as an author (ghost authorship).

The best approach is to negotiate clear expectations for the roles of student and professor with regard to course work and writing for publication. If the student is expected to complete a project for course credit, the teacher should evaluate the work for a grade first, and then discuss the work necessary to author a manuscript for publication. At that time, the relative contributions of each person to the manuscript can be negotiated, and authorship credit can be assigned fairly. As a general rule, a student is listed as first author on any multiple-authored manuscript that is substantially based on the student's thesis or dissertation (American Psychological Association [APA], 1994).

COPYRIGHT

Copyright is a form of legal protection to the authors of "original works of authorship," including literary, dramatic, musical, artistic, and other intellectual works, preventing others from copying them (U.S. Copyright Office, 1999). U.S. copyright law is defined by the Copyright Act of 1976. Copyright provides protection for any original material created by the author, including both published and unpublished works. Co-authors of papers written collaboratively have equal rights to the copyright.

The copyright law gives authors, or whomever holds the copyright, five exclusive rights: (1) reproduction, (2) modification, (3) publication, (4) performance, and (5) public display of the work (U.S. Copyright Office, 1999). The owner of the copyright is the only person allowed to exercise these five rights; anyone else who wants to reproduce, modify, publish, perform, or display the work must get permission from the copyright owner.

Protected Works

Copyright protects original works "that are fixed in a tangible form of expression" (U.S. Copyright Office, 2000a, p. 7). These protected works include the following:

- Literary works (eg, articles, books, journals, computer programs, and digital formats)
- Musical works including the accompanying words
- Dramatic works including the accompanying music
- Pantomimes and choreographic works
- Pictorial, graphic, and sculptural works
- Motion pictures and other audiovisual works
- Sound recordings
- Architectural works.

For works created since 1978, the term of protection for copyright is the life of the author plus 70 years. For works created between 1964 and 1977, the protection for copyright is 28 years for the original term plus an automatic 67-year renewal; for materials created between 1923 and 1963, the protection extends for the original 28-year term with an additional 67 years if the copyright was renewed. Works created before 1923 are in the public domain.

Unprotected Works

Several categories of materials, though, are not protected by copyright, including the following (U.S. Copyright Office, 1999):

- Works that have not been fixed in a tangible form of expression, such as speeches or performances that have not been written or recorded
- Titles, names, short phrases, and slogans; familiar symbols or designs; variations of typographic ornamentation, lettering, or coloring; and listings of ingredients or contents
- Ideas, procedures, methods, systems, processes, concepts, principles, discoveries, or devices, as distinguished from a description, explana-

tion, or illustration. Although the ideas may not be protected by copyright law, the written description of the ideas may be.

- Works consisting entirely of information that is common property and has no original authorship, for instance, calendars and lists or tables taken from public documents or other common sources
- U.S. government works
- Material that has fallen into the public domain.

U.S. Copyright Office

Information about copyright is available to authors through the U.S Copyright Office at the following address:

U.S. Copyright Office
Library of Congress
101 Independence Ave. S.E.
Washington, DC 20559-6000

Frequently requested circulars, regulations, and other related materials and copyright application forms also are available through the Internet at *http://lcweb.loc.gov/copyright*.

Transfer of Copyright

The copyright is held initially by the author, or co-authors, of the manuscript. When a manuscript is being considered for publication by a journal, each author contributing to the paper typically transfers the copyright to the publisher either at the time the manuscript is submitted or when it is accepted. Publishers usually require assignment of the copyright to them so that they in turn may publish the article and distribute it in different forms. If the copyright transfer form is submitted with the manuscript before its acceptance by the journal, the copyright reverts to the author, or co-authors, if the manuscript is not published.

Publishers have their own copyright transfer forms, which are signed by each author. Figure 4-1 provides an example of the copyright transfer form from *MCN, The American Journal of Maternal/Child Nursing*. When the copyright is transferred, the publisher becomes the legal owner of the published paper. Neither the author nor others may reproduce the paper without written approval of the copyright holder—the publisher.

Authors who want to reproduce any figure, table, or text from the copyrighted material must receive permission from the copyright holder. This is

MCN, The American Journal of Maternal/Child Nursing
Authorship Responsibility, Financial Disclosure, and Copyright Transfer

Manuscript Title:

Corresponding Author:

Address, Telephone, and Fax Numbers:

Each author must read and sign the following statements and, if necessary, photocopy this document and distribute to coauthors for their original ink signatures. Please compile all forms and include them with this manuscript.

CONDITIONS OF SUBMISSION:
RETAINED RIGHTS: Other than copyright, all proprietary rights (such as patent rights) are retained by the authors.
ORIGINALITY: The authors warrant that this submission is an original work. Neither this work nor a similar work has been published or will be submitted for publication elsewhere while under consideration by this Journal.
AUTHORSHIP RESPONSIBILITY: The authors certify that they have participated sufficiently in the intellectual content, the analysis of data, if applicable, and the writing of the work, to take public responsibility for it. They have reviewed the final version of the work, believe it represents valid work and approve it for publication. Moreover, should the editors of the Journal request the data upon which the work is based, they shall produce it.
DISCLAIMER: The undersigned warrant that this work contains no libelous or unlawful statements and does not infringe on the rights of others. If excerpts (text or figures) from copyrighted works are included, written permission will be secured by the authors prior to submission, and credit will be properly acknowledged.

INSTITUTIONAL REVIEW BOARD/ANIMAL CARE COMMITTEE APPROVAL:
The undersigned authors certify that their institutions have approved the protocol for any investigation involving humans or animals and that all experimentation was conducted in conformity with ethical and humane principles of research.

TRANSFER OF COPYRIGHT:
AUTHORS' OWN WORK: The undersigned authors hereby transfer, assign, or otherwise convey all copyright ownership worldwide, in all languages, and in all forms of media now or hereafter known, including electronic media such as CD-ROM, Internet, and Intranet, to Lippincott Williams & Wilkins, Inc., in the event that such work is accepted for publication in the Journal. To reproduce any figure or text from this article in future works of their own, the authors must obtain written permission. Such permission will not be unreasonably withheld by the copyright holder.

Figure 4-1. Copyright transfer form.

GOVERNMENT EMPLOYEES:
*If this article exists in the public domain because it was written as part of the official duties of the Authors as employees of the U.S. government, check this box. ☐
Note to Government Employees: If this work has been written in the course of employment by the United States Government, the above box should be checked, and a copy of the relevant departmental statement of policy attached. A work prepared by a government employee as part of his/her official duties is called a "work of the U.S. Government" and is not subject to copyright. If it is not prepared as part of the employee's official duties, it may be copyrighted.

FINANCIAL DISCLOSURE:
The undersigned authors certify that they have no commercial associations (eg, consultancies, stock ownership, equity interest, patent-licensing arrangements, etc.) that might pose a conflict of interest in connection with the submitted article, except as disclosed on a separate attachment. All funding sources supporting the work and all institutional or corporate affiliations of the authors are acknowledged in a footnote.

Signature _____	Printed Name _____	Date _____
☐ Author's own work	☐ Work for hire	☐ Government
Signature _____	Printed Name _____	Date _____
☐ Author's own work	☐ Work for hire	☐ Government
Signature _____	Printed Name _____	Date _____
☐ Author's own work	☐ Work for hire	☐ Government
Signature _____	Printed Name _____	Date _____
☐ Author's own work	☐ Work for hire	☐ Government

Figure 4-1. *Continued.*

true even for the author's own article because the copyright was transferred to and is then held by the publisher. This principle is clear in the Transfer of Copyright section in Figure 4-1.

Copying and Reproducing Copyrighted Material

The fair use provisions of the copyright law, contained in Title 17 of the United States Code, Section 107, allow the author to quote, copy, or reproduce a small amount of text from a copyrighted work without permission of the publisher or other holder of the copyright. Fair use of copyrighted materials for purposes such as teaching, scholarship, and research is not considered an infringement of copyright. If it is more than a small section of copyrighted work, though, the author needs to get written permission from the copyright holder to use the material. Fair use does not give authors permission to reproduce complete articles or to republish one of their articles published in a different journal.

In determining fair use, four factors are considered (U.S. Copyright Office, 2000b, p. 16):

1. Purpose of the use, including whether it is for commercial purposes or for nonprofit educational purposes
2. Nature of the copyrighted work
3. Amount of the material copied and how substantial it is in relation to the copyrighted work as a whole
4. Effect of the use on the potential market for or value of the copyrighted work.

The amount of text subject to fair use is based on the proportion to the whole, but this proportion is not determined by number of words (AMA, 1998, p. 124). There is no specific word length in the copyright law that is acceptable. Therefore, the author needs to consider these four factors when questioning whether permission should be obtained from the copyright holder. Some publishers may specify the number of words that are allowed to be reproduced without written permission. For example, the APA provides guidelines for authors as to the extent of text and number of tables and figures that may be reproduced without written permission from APA and from the author of the reproduced article published in an APA journal (APA, 1994).

The author should be careful to include the reference to the original source. Any direct quotations should be placed in quotation marks or indented to set off the quoted material, again with a reference to the original source.

Permission should be obtained for quotations that extend for a few paragraphs. The AMA (1998) suggested that the length quoted should not diminish the "value of the original work" (p. 124). Entire tables, figures, and illustrations may not be reproduced without permission. This includes use of a table, figure, or other type of graphic in a paper prepared for a course. Using one or two sentences from a table would be acceptable if the original source is referenced, but reprinting the entire table is not. Authors should obtain permission to reprint and adapt tables, figures, and illustrations for a manuscript and for other types of writing projects.

Materials on Internet

These same principles apply for materials published on the Internet. Articles and other materials published on the Internet may be copied only if the information is created by the federal government, the copyright has expired, or the copyright has been abandoned by the holder (Valette, 2000). Works published on the Internet are not automatically in the public domain. With rapidly changing technology and more on-line publishing, the author should consult experts with questions about whether permission is needed for reproducing materials from the Internet and other electronic forms of publication.

PERMISSIONS

In obtaining permission to reprint previously published material in a manuscript, the author should make this request early in the writing process to avoid delays in the submission of the manuscript. Permission letters are needed before the article is published, but journals may request that they be included when the manuscript is submitted.

For journal articles, which usually are copyrighted by the publisher of the journal, the author should write to the publisher requesting permission to reproduce the selection of text, table, figure, or other illustration in the manuscript. Information on how to obtain permission from the publisher, with the address and other contact information for its permissions department, often is included in the masthead or Information for Authors page in the journal. For a book, the copyright holder is specified on the page after the title page. When the authors of the original works hold the copyrights, they would grant permission to reprint their material and would be contacted directly.

The author may check the Copyright Clearance Center, which provides licensing systems for the reproduction and distribution of copyrighted materials in print and electronic formats. The Copyright Clearance Center manages the rights for many copyrighted works, for publishers, and for authors (Copyright Clearance Center, 2000). The Copyright Clearance Center may be reached at

Copyright Clearance Center
222 Rosewood Drive
Danvers, MA 01923 USA
URL http://www.copyright.com/Contact.html.

Permissions Letter

An example of a letter requesting permission to reprint copyrighted materials is presented in Display 4.1. In the letter, the author should include the complete citation of the original work; a description of the material to be reprinted, such as portion of the text, table, figure, or other illustration including the page numbers where it can be found; publication in which the material will be used; and how the original work would be adapted. For books, the publisher typically provides a permission form for the author to use for requesting permissions to reprint.

DISPLAY 4.1	**Sample Permissions Letter**

Permissions Department
Lippincott Williams & Wilkins
530 Walnut Street
Philadelphia, PA 19106

Dear Permissions Department:

I am requesting permission to include Figure 1. Instructional software evaluation form (pp. 146–148) in a manuscript that I am writing. The manuscript, "Integrating Computer Programs in Clinical Teaching in Nursing," will be submitted to the *Journal of Nursing Education* or a similar scholarly journal. The figure was published in Boyce, B.A., & Winne, M.D. (2000). Developing an evaluation tool for instructional software programs. *Nurse Educator, 25,* 145–148.

Thank you for your consideration of this request.

Sincerely,

[Author's name, credentials
Complete mailing address
Fax number and other contact information]

Conditions

The copyright holder may require certain conditions when granting permission to use the material, for instance, using a specific credit line and copyright statement. Display 4.2 provides examples of how to state an adaptation of an original work and sample credit lines.

The author may incur a permission fee when requesting copyright permission. If the secondary use of the material is for commercial purposes, the fee may be significant (AMA, 1998, p. 127). Another possibility is that permission to reprint may not be granted.

Photographs

Patients, nurses, and other persons shown in photographs need to provide written permission for reproduction of the photograph in the manuscript. In the letter asking their permission, the author should include the title of the manuscript, possible journal in which it might be published, and when the photograph was taken. The subject in the photograph must give a signed consent, which the author in turn submits with the manuscript.

Sample Permissions Credit Lines

REPRINTED WITH PERMISSION

Figure 1. HRQOL conceptual model developed by Wilson and Cleary (1995). Reprinted with permission, *JAMA*, 273, 59–65. Copyright 1995, American Medical Association.

Figure 2. Clinical evaluation instrument. Copyright 2000, K. Smith. Reproduced with permission.

Table 1. Roles of teacher and student in discussion. From: Gaberson, K.B., & Oermann, M.H. (1999). *Clinical teaching strategies in nursing.* New York: Springer, 169. Copyright 1999, Springer. Reprinted with permission.

ADAPTED FROM

Table 1 is adapted from: O'Farrell, P., Murray, J., & Hotz, S.B. (2000). Psychologic distress among spouses of patients undergoing cardiac rehabilitation. *Heart & Lung, 29,* 97–104.

 ## HOW MANY IS TOO MANY?

The author needs to avoid writing several manuscripts when one would be sufficient. Each paper should make its own contribution to the literature and should not overlap with one already published. Editors deserve to publish original papers, and readers assume that what they are reading in their journals are original ideas.

Whereas some projects lend themselves to writing more than one paper, others do not. An example of dividing a research study into separate manuscripts when one would suffice is provided by a study on the effectiveness of pressure ulcer treatments. In the study, the researcher collected data on clinical outcomes such as the location, stage, and size of the ulcer; hours of nursing care each patient received and level of education of nursing staff; and treatment costs. Separate manuscripts would not be appropriate in presenting the findings of this research because the author measured the effectiveness of the treatments based on clinical outcomes, staff variables, and cost. These measures are closely related and as a whole describe the treatments' effectiveness.

Some research studies and other projects, though, may be divided legitimately into more than one manuscript. The author may report the findings of research in one journal and a critical analysis of the literature in another. The implications of the findings for nursing practice even may be reported in yet a third article, as long as each of the manuscripts has a clear message and presents new information—not what has appeared in the other articles.

When writing about a clinical project or an innovation in practice, a professional issue, and other nonresearch topics, the same question should be asked: Is it legitimate to divide the topic into separate manuscripts, or would one suffice? The author may be planning to write a manuscript about nursing care for patients treated with a new surgical procedure that has been initiated recently in the clinical setting. Separate manuscripts about care of these patients in the immediate postoperative period and home care would be inappropriate. The care of these patients would be better presented across the continuum, and neither manuscript would be so long as to warrant separate papers.

Duplicate or Redundant Publication

The publication of essentially the same material in two or more publications is termed duplicate or redundant publication. Duplicate publication can range from disseminating the same content in different forms to different audiences to submitting duplicate manuscripts with identical content to different publishers (Blancett, Flanagin, & Young, 1995). The ethical issues associated with duplicate publication are wasteful use of resources and originality of scientific work. When an author submits the same material to two or more journals simultaneously or attempts to divide one work into several publications, the resources of scientific publication are used inappropriately. The time and energy of peer reviewers and editors and the financial resources of publishers are invested in reviewing and preparing manuscripts for publication. A manuscript cannot be published in more than one journal because of copyright considerations; when the manuscript is accepted for publication in one journal and the author must withdraw it from consideration by others, those resources are wasted, contributing to the ever-increasing costs of scientific publication (Duncan, 1999; Rogers, 1999).

Publishers, editors, and readers of scientific papers assume that published material is original. Therefore, editors typically require authors of manuscripts to certify that their submitted manuscripts are not under consideration for publication elsewhere, and that if accepted for publication, the material would not be published elsewhere in the same form without the consent of the editors (Day, 1998).

Duplicate publication can take the form of shotgunning or salami slicing. Each practice has associated ethical issues.

Shotgunning

Shotgunning is submitting the same manuscript for review by two or more journals. An author who engages in shotgunning typically intends to wait until the manuscript is accepted for publication by one journal, and then withdraw it from consideration by others. However, the author has no control over the timing of review procedures, and at worst, this practice could lead to publication of the same material in more than one journal, violating the standard of originality of scientific publication. At a minimum, the author has inconvenienced the editor and reviewers of the journal from which the manu-script was withdrawn.

Shotgunning may be sanctioned as an inappropriate act according to the Uniform Requirements or specific journal policy. The Uniform Requirements suggest that if duplicate publication occurs, a notice of redundant publication be published by the journal editor with or without the author's explanation or approval (ICMJE, 1997). Additional sanctions also may apply. If an author publishes two identical articles, a journal may prohibit the author from submitting a manuscript to the journal for a specified period of time.

Salami Slicing

Salami slicing (divided or fragmented publication) is the practice of breaking down findings from a single research study or project into a series of papers (known as "least publishable units") submitted to different journals or to the same journal at different times. The intent of salami slicing usually is to increase the number of publications attributable to an author. Some editors do not regard salami slicing as an ethical violation (Rogers, 1999); others do, citing it as an example of wasteful publication and an abuse of scientific publication (Blancett, 1991; Huth, 1986).

Divided publication can obscure the true value of the findings of a research study, making them appear more important than they really are; they may confound meta-analyses of research findings; and they may misrepresent the true incidence of reported phenomena. For example, Davidhizar, Bechtel, and McEwen (1999) pointed out that publication of similar information about cultural differences in more than one journal may blur the distinction between original research and secondary analysis and may lead to overgeneralization of implications for interventions, which may adversely affect the health outcomes of already exploited populations.

Acceptable Duplicate Publication

Duplicate publication does not include sending a manuscript rejected by one journal to another. When a manuscript is returned to the author, it then may be submitted to another journal for review. Other forms of publication not considered redundant by the ICMJE (1997) are manuscripts that follow preliminary reports as abstracts or poster presentations, manuscripts presented at professional conferences that are published in the proceedings, and press reports.

The key to whether duplicate publication is acceptable is disclosure (Blancett, 1991; Blancett, Flanagin, & Young, 1995). It is unethical when authors do not notify editors about duplicate publications and do not include references to them. Authors should inform editors about duplicate publications, and copies of these articles should be sent with the submission. If there is any question about whether a manuscript reflects duplicate publication, the author should include a statement to the editor describing similar work. The ICMJE (1997) recommended alerting the editor if the manuscript is based on the same subjects as in an earlier publication. Earlier articles always should be referenced in a subsequent manuscript in both the text and reference list. Some journals such as *Applied Nursing Research* ask authors to specify any publication in which the same content or data set has been used and how the submitted manuscript differs.

Secondary Publication

Secondary publication is the republication or parallel publication of an article in more than one journal with consent of the involved editors (AMA, 1998, p. 99). An example of a secondary publication is when an article is translated for publication in a journal of a different language than the original. Typically, secondary publications are released at least 1 week after the primary publication, are intended for a different audience than the original paper, do not modify the data or conclusions of the original paper, and include a footnote on the title page that informs readers that the paper was previously published (ICMJE, 1997). The footnote should contain the full reference to the primary paper.

 ACCURACY

"Responsible dissemination of scholarly work is a critical aspect of maintaining scientific integrity within a profession" (Clark, 1993, p. 113). Readers assume the truth of published material and hold authors accountable for ensuring accuracy (Cormach, 1994). Standards for disseminating scholarly work include reporting of valid data and avoiding the publication of fraudulent, false, or fabricated data. Examples of fraudulent reporting include fabrication of data and selective reporting by omission of conflicting data (Clark, 1993).

False data may be disseminated by means other than deliberate fraud. Careless researchers and authors may make mistakes through lack of rigor or discipline, such as mishandling of data, failure to supervise research assistants or to edit manuscript drafts carefully, or creating systematic bias in the design of a study. Such errors are not ethical violations, but they raise concerns about the competence of researchers and writers (Clark, 1993). Errors that are discovered by the author after publication should be brought to the attention of the editor so that a correction notice can be published (APA, 1994).

Errors in accuracy of published material range from the serious (eg, a significant omission in the description of a treatment) to the merely annoying (eg, an incomplete or incorrect reference citation). Authors should carefully check the accuracy of cited sources and proofread drafts, edited manuscripts, and typeset proofs for errors introduced by others involved in the publication process (Cormach, 1994). When possible, authors should cite primary sources of information, and they should never cite sources they have not personally read. In a review of 262 articles published in nursing journals, Taylor (1998) found an overall citation error rate of 45.8%; 39.3% of references contained at least one significant error. Schulmeister's (1998) findings were similar, with 32% of the sampled articles from three nursing journals containing citation errors serious enough that the cited works could not be retrieved. One inaccurate reference citation can lead to many others if careless authors copy the erroneous citation without verifying its accuracy. Multiple cross-references of this sort may prevent the correct original source from being identified, requiring the use of secondary sources of information. To prevent such problems, authors should read and cite original sources of information when possible and judge the accuracy of all references cited (Davidhizar, 1999).

 ## PLAGIARISM

A quotation is the use of the exact words of another, indicated by quotation marks. Paraphrasing refers to summarizing content, rearranging the order of words, or changing some words from source material (APA, 1994). Many writers, especially students, believe that plagiarism refers only to failure to indicate and cite properly a verbatim quotation. However, any time authors present the ideas of another as their own without giving proper credit to the source, plagiarism has occurred. Vogelsang (1997) suggested that using materials from an original source without appropriate attribution of credit is an act of professional theft and deception. Using ideas and information from sources not cited shows lack of respect and regard for the original author's knowledge and the efforts that were applied to the publication of those ideas (Vogelsang, 1997).

Plagiarism can be considered a crime of theft of intellectual property. It is not a victimless crime; plagiarism can harm the author of the original source material, the scientific community, and the plagiarizer. Outcomes of well-publicized cases of discovered plagiarism include public humiliation and damaged reputations, letters of reprimand, withholding or loss of academic degrees, termination of employment, and lawsuits (Vogelsang, 1997).

Peer reviewers and members of editorial boards are guilty of plagiarism if they use ideas and information found in the manuscripts they review for their own gain (Clark, 1993). For example, peer reviewers might recommend rejection of a manuscript but incorporate ideas from the manuscript in their own writings; this, too, is plagiarism. This is discussed later in the chapter under Conflict of Interest.

Plagiarism is fairly easy to prove if a writer uses verbatim or nearly identical copy of material published by someone else, but it is more difficult to detect if the form of the material has been altered, for example, by changes in wording (Cormach, 1994). The ultimate test of whether plagiarism has occurred is to compare the new material with the original source (Vogelsang, 1997). Authors can avoid plagiarism through adequate and appropriate documentation, but sometimes this is not easy to do. All authors absorb and use the ideas of others, and a writer may forget the original source of an idea or even that there was an original source. However, unless authors specifically acknowledge the sources of ideas, they claim credit for them (AMA, 1998, p. 89; Clark, 1993). It sometimes is difficult to make a distinction between matters of general knowledge, which do not require documentation, and sources of information that do, or to separate plagiarism of ideas from general influences on thought. It has been suggested that information that occurs in five or more sources may be considered general knowledge (Clark, 1993). However, it usually is better to include too much information about sources of information than too little (AMA, 1998, p. 89).

Can an author plagiarize unintentionally? In some cases, it is unclear whether the author lacked knowledge about proper documentation of sources or whether intentional plagiarism occurred, especially with student authors. However, ignorance of the meaning of plagiarism is not an acceptable excuse for such misconduct (Clark, 1993). Skillful paraphrasing without plagiarizing requires the writer to understand and synthesize the material from the original source so that the resulting copy moves beyond the use of synonyms and altered sentence structure (Vogelsang, 1997).

Copying of one's own previously published material without proper citation of source also is an example of plagiarism. Remember that once a publisher holds a copyright for published material, that material cannot be reused without permission from the copyright holder, even by the original author of the material. Even short verbatim quotes from an author's previously published content should be referenced back to the original source, using appropriate citation style, and the author should seek permission from the copyright holder to reuse lengthier portions. If an author plans to publish ideas similar to those in previously published works, but in a completely different form, the editor of the original publication should be consulted as a courtesy. If the author holds the copyright, the author may reuse material freely (eg, a theory, model, or research tool), but the work should not be represented as original material in more than one publication (Clark, 1993).

CONFLICT OF INTEREST

To facilitate readers' determination of the accuracy and value of published works, authors must disclose any financial or other competing interest that might cast doubt on their impartiality. Does the author or the affiliated institution or business stand to gain financially from the mention of a commercial product in a publication? If so, questions may arise about whether this financial interest has affected the study results (Clark, 1993). If the writer holds stock in a company whose products are promoted in the publication, the writer has an obligation to disclose this association to the editor, who then has a duty to inform readers. Similarly, if a researcher received grant support for a study, the source of the funding should be reported in any published research report so that readers may determine if the content of the research report relates to the potential vested interest of the funding agency (Blancett, 1991).

When an author includes personal opinions or prejudiced language, especially in a research report, this writing style raises questions about the writer's motives and scientific impartiality. "Controversial issues must be presented fairly, without animosity" (Carpenito, 1998, p. 3). Authors should be able to interpret and report their own beliefs with as little bias as possible, focusing on practical scientific consequences of knowledge with no deliberate misinterpretation. Objectivity in reporting and writing is closely linked to the ways in which knowledge is gained and disseminated in any discipline (Crigger, 1998).

Likewise, peer reviewers must disclose any prior bias for or against an author or the ideas presented in a manuscript. Blind or masked (APA, 1994) review processes are designed to reduce such bias by protecting the identity of both the author and the peer reviewer. If the peer reviewer has a favorable opinion of an author, blind review protects the discipline by focusing the evaluation on the author's ideas. If the peer reviewer has an unfavorable opinion of an author, blind review protects the writer from this negative bias. However, sometimes it is possible for reviewers to discern the identity of a writer, particularly if the author writes in a highly specialized field (Crigger, 1998) or has extensive prior publications that are cited in the manuscript under review. A reviewer who suspects the identity of an author or who is aware of negative or positive bias toward the ideas expressed in the manuscript should report this potential conflict to the editor, who then may seek another reviewer for that manuscript. Because the peer review process protects the author's identity in most cases, it is difficult for reviewers to detect ghost authorship (Larkin, 1999).

However, bias toward or against certain ideas may be inherent in the process of choosing peer reviewers because they are appointed by an editor or editorial board and not elected or randomly selected. The assumption underlying selection of peer reviewers is that expertise in a subject area assures fairness in reviewing manuscripts in that area. The validity of that assumption may be questionable, since experts hold established beliefs about their specific content areas that strongly influence how they receive new and conflicting ideas. In fact, expert reviewers may be more biased than individuals with less experience in their content areas. Content bias is more likely to occur in situations where there are few reviewers or if certain reviewers always are assigned to review manuscripts in specific content areas (reviewer monopolies) (Crigger, 1998).

PROTECTING THE RIGHTS OF INDIVIDUALS IN PUBLICATIONS

In preparing a manuscript, the author needs to protect the rights of individuals to privacy and to avoid harming the reputations of others by defamation.

Privacy Rights

Publications in nursing, medicine, and other health care disciplines must protect the rights of certain individuals to privacy. Historically, this effort has included omitting patient names, initials, and case numbers from published case reports; removing identifying information from x-ray films, digital images, and laboratory slides; deleting certain identifying details from descriptions of patients or participants in research studies; and concealing certain facial features of patients in published photographs (eg, placing black bars over the eyes). However, masking facial features does not always disguise identities sufficiently, and since the late 1980s, its use has not been recommended. If written informed consent to publish a photographic likeness has not been obtained from a patient or legally authorized representative, the photograph should not be published (AMA, 1998, pp. 141–142). Authors who have obtained such written consents should include them with other permissions when the manuscript is submitted.

To prevent patients and participants in research studies from recognizing descriptions of themselves in published reports, some authors omit certain descriptive data from the manuscript, including age, sex, and occupation. However, omitting such details may hinder future investigations and meta-analyses. For example, occupational information might be useful to a researcher who is conducting a study of occupational injuries. Altering some demographic details about patients or research participants may appear to be a harmless way to protect the identities of these individuals, but doing so allows falsified data to be published—a serious breach of scientific integrity (ICMJE, 1997). Altered or falsified data also can affect a subsequent investigation or meta-analysis, for example, changing the name of a city can contribute error to an epidemiologic analysis of disease outbreak locations (AMA, 1998, pp. 141–142). The Uniform Requirements suggest that identifying information about patients should not be published unless it is essential for scientific purposes and that the patient or legally authorized representative should be allowed to review the manuscript before giving informed consent for the information to be published (ICMJE,1997).

Defamation

Although every citizen is guaranteed freedom of expression by the First Amendment to the Constitution of the United States, this right is balanced against the right to protect one's personal reputation. Therefore, authors, editors, and publishers must take care to not harm the reputations of others by defamation, thereby exposing them to public ridicule, contempt, hatred, or financial loss. Defamation can take the form of libel or slander, but it always includes a false public statement concerning another (AMA, 1998, p. 143).

Libel is a false statement about another living person or existing entity, made in print, writing, images, or signs. In some states, malicious intent is required to prove libel (AMA, 1998, pp. 143–147; Cormach, 1994). Slander is defamation by oral expression or gestures; with the increasing use of digital publication, including mixtures of print, audio, and video content, the distinction between libel and slander has become increasingly blurred (AMA, 1998, p. 143).

The laws concerning defamation are complex, and it is beyond the scope of this book to offer specific advice about how to avoid defamation in the process of writing for publication. Authors are advised to consult the editors of the publications to which they submit manuscripts for specific guidance.

SUMMARY

Ethical and legal issues affecting writing for publication include authorship, copyright, duplicate publication, accuracy, plagiarism, conflict of interest, and protecting the rights of those involved in the publication process. This chapter provides an overview of these issues and offers suggestions for preventing or minimizing ethical and legal problems related to writing for publication.

Ethical issues of unjustified, irresponsible, and incomplete authorship center around the question of who is entitled to be listed as the author of a scientific publication. The listing of many author names on a short paper suggests the inclusion of some individuals who do not qualify for authorship. However, irresponsible authorship reaches beyond the number of authors listed; related issues include giving authorship credit to individuals who made only trivial contributions to published manuscripts, if any (guest or honorary authorship) or not listing as an author one who actually wrote part or all of the manuscript (ghost authorship). Faculty members who co-author papers with students should take care to clearly identify the differences between giving guidance in the role of teacher and assuming the role of author.

Copyright is a form of legal protection to the authors of "original works of authorship." Because copyright is a form of property, it can be assigned to another. Authors own their manuscripts until they sign a copyright transfer form, which then transfers the ownership to the publisher. This gives the publisher the right to reproduce, modify, publish, perform, and publicly display the work. Authors who want to reproduce any figure, table, or text from the copyrighted material must receive permission from the copyright holder. This is true even for the author's own article because the copyright was transferred to and then is held by the publisher. The publication of essentially the same material in two or more publications is termed duplicate, redundant, or wasteful publication. When an author submits the same material to more than one journal or attempts to divide one work into several publications, the resources of scientific publication are used inappropriately.

Readers assume the truth of published material, and authors are accountable for ensuring accuracy. Standards for disseminating scholarly work include reporting of valid data and avoiding the publication of fraudulent, false, or fabricated data. False data may be disseminated because of carelessness in addition to deliberate fraud. Authors should carefully check the accuracy of cited sources and proofread drafts, edited manuscripts, and typeset proofs for errors introduced at any stage of the publication process. When possible, authors should cite primary sources of information, and they should never cite sources they have not personally read. One inaccurate reference citation can lead to many others if careless authors copy the erroneous citation without verifying its accuracy.

A related issue is plagiarism, the act of presenting the ideas of another as one's own without giving proper credit to their source. Many writers, especially students, believe that plagiarism refers only to failure to indicate and cite properly a verbatim quotation, but plagiarism also can involve paraphrasing without citing the source of the ideas. Peer reviewers and members of editorial boards commit plagiarism if they use ideas and information found in the manuscripts they review for their own gain. Authors can plagiarize unintentionally if they lack knowledge about proper documentation of sources, but ignorance of the meaning of plagiarism is not an acceptable excuse for such misconduct.

To allow readers to determine the accuracy and value of published works, authors must disclose any financial or other competing interest that might cast doubt on their impartiality. If the author or affiliated employer or business stand to gain financially from the mention of a commercial product in a publication, questions may arise about whether this financial interest has affected the study results. If the writer has a financial interest in a company whose products are promoted in the publication, the writer has an obligation to disclose this association to the editor, who then has a duty to inform readers. Similarly, if a researcher receives grant support for a study, the source of the funding should be reported in any published research report.

Objectivity in writing is related to the ways in which knowledge is gained and disseminated. Inclusion of personal opinions or prejudiced language in a manuscript invites questions about the writer's motives and scientific impartiality.

Other ethical and legal issues involved in writing for publication relate to protecting the rights of individuals. Publications in health care disciplines must protect the right to privacy of patients and participants in research projects. Patients should give consent for publication of identifying information about themselves after reviewing the manuscript to be submitted for publication.

Freedom of expression is balanced against the right to protect one's personal reputation. Therefore, authors, editors, and publishers must take care to not defame the reputations of others, thereby exposing them to public ridicule or financial loss. Defamation always involves a false public statement concerning another and can take the form of libel or slander. Libel is a false statement about another living person or existing entity made in print, writing, images, or signs. Slander is defamation by oral expression or gestures; the increasing use of digital publication that includes mixtures of print, audio, and video content has blurred the distinction between libel and slander. Because the laws concerning defamation are complex, authors are advised to consult the editors of the publications to which they submit manuscripts for specific guidance about how to avoid defamation.

REFERENCES

American Medical Association. (1998). *Manual of style: A guide for authors and editors* (9th ed.). Baltimore: Lippincott Williams & Wilkins.

American Psychological Association. (1994). *Publication manual of the American Psychological Association* (4th ed.). Washington, DC: APA.

Blancett, S.S. (1991). The ethics of writing and publishing. *Journal of Nursing Administration, 21*(5), 31–36.

Blancett, S.S., Flanagin, A., & Young, R.K. (1995). Duplicate publication in the nursing literature. *Image: Journal of Nursing Scholarship, 27*(1), 51–56.

Butler, L., & Ginn, D. (1998). Canadian nurses' views on assignment of publication credit for scholarly and scientific work. *Canadian Journal of Nursing Research, 30,* 171–183.

Carpenito, L. (1998). In search of the truth or Jerry Springer. *Nursing Forum, 33*(2), 3.

Clark, A.J. (1993). Responsible dissemination of scholarly work. *Journal of Neuroscience Nursing, 25,* 113–117.

Copyright Clearance Center. (2000). Creating copyright solutions. [On-line]. Available: *http://www.copyright.com/About/default.html.* Accessed May 24, 2000.

Cormach, D. (1994). *Writing for health care professionals.* London: Blackwell.

Crigger, N.J. (1998). What we owe the author: Rethinking editorial peer review. *Nursing Ethics, 5,* 451–458.

Davidhizar, R., Bechtel, G.A., & McEwen, M. (1999). Referencing in transcultural nursing: An ethical analysis. *Nursing Forum, 34*(4), 14–18.

Day, R.A. (1998). *How to write and publish a scientific paper.* Phoenix, AZ: Oryx Press.

Duncan, A.M. (1999). Authorship, dissemination of research findings, and related matters. *Applied Nursing Research, 12,* 101–106.

Gaeta, T.J. (1999). Authorship: "Law" and order. *Academic Emergency Medicine, 6,* 297–301.

Garfield, E. (1995). Giving credit only where it is due: The problem of defining authorship. *The Scientist, 9*(19), 13.

Huth, E.J. (1986). Irresponsible authorship and wasteful publication. *Annals of Internal Medicine, 104,* 257–259.

International Committee of Medical Journal Editors. (1997). Uniform requirements for manuscripts submitted to biomedical journals. *Annals of Internal Medicine, 126,* 36–47. Also available: *http://www.icmje.org/.*

Larkin, M. (1999). Whose article is it anyway? *The Lancet, 354,* 136.

Rennie, D., & Flanagin, A. (1994). Authorship! Authorship! Guests, ghosts, grafters, and the two-sided coin. *Journal of the American Medical Association, 271,* 469–471.

Rogers, L.F. (1999). Salami slicing, shotgunning, and the ethics of authorship. *American Journal of Roentgenology, 173,* 265.

Schulmeister, L. (1998). Quotation and reference accuracy of three nursing journals. *Image, 30,* 143–146.

Taylor, M.K. (1998). The practical effects of errors in reference lists in nursing research journals. *Nursing Research, 47,* 300–303.

U.S. Copyright Office. (1999). Copyright basics. [On-line]. Available: *http://www.loc.gov/copyright/circs/circ1.html#wci.* Accessed May 23, 2000.

U.S. Copyright Office. (2000a). Title 17 of the United States Code. Sec. 102. Subject matter of copyright: In general (p. 7). [On-line]. Available: *http://www.loc.gov/copyright/title17/chapter01.pdf.* Accessed May 24, 2000.

U.S. Copyright Office. (2000b). Title 17 of the United States Code. Sec. 107. Limitations on exclusive rights: Fair use (p. 16). [On-line]. Available: *http://www.loc.gov/copyright/title17/chapter01.pdf.* Accessed May 23, 2000.

Valette, R. (2000). What is copyright protection? [On-line]. Available: *http://whatiscopyright.org.* Accessed May 24, 2000.

Vogelsang, J. (1997). Plagiarism: An act of stealing. *Journal of Perianesthesia Nursing, 12,* 422–425.

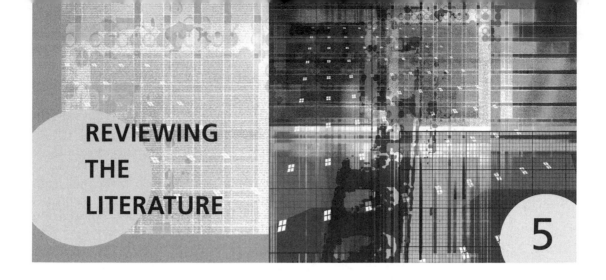

REVIEWING THE LITERATURE

5

Conducting a literature review is a skill the author needs to develop to be an effective writer. Often, before writing the manuscript, the author has reviewed, critiqued, and synthesized the literature as a basis for a research study, an innovation, or a project to be described in the paper. In this situation, the literature may need to be updated, or if the focus of the manuscript is on the implications of the study for clinical practice, another review of the literature from this perspective may be helpful. Other times, though, the author begins with a topic to be considered for a manuscript but has not yet searched the literature. The review enables the author to decide if the manuscript is worth writing in the first place and gives the author an understanding of material that has already been published on the topic. Either way, the author cannot begin writing without completing a review of the literature.

This chapter prepares the author for conducting and writing a literature review for a manuscript. Although literature reviews for research studies, theses and dissertations, course work, and clinical projects vary in the types of literature used, their comprehensiveness, and how they are summarized for the reader, the process of reviewing the literature is the same. This chapter also describes bibliographic databases useful for literature reviews in nursing, how to select databases, search strategies, analyzing and synthesizing the literature, and writing the literature review for a manuscript and other types of papers. The goal here is to enable the reader to develop skill in conducting literature reviews for writing papers in nursing.

PURPOSES OF LITERATURE REVIEW

A literature review is a critique and summary of current knowledge about a topic, for research and for use in clinical practice, teaching, administration, and other areas of nursing. There are three main purposes of reviewing the literature. The first purpose is to describe what is known already about a topic. The literature review provides the background for designing a research study, answering questions about clinical practice, developing new projects, and making other decisions in nursing. It reveals existing knowledge about a topic and related areas.

The literature search also lets the author decide whether to write the paper. The author may have an idea to share with readers but may find from the review of the literature that the topic already has been adequately covered and another article is unnecessary. The opposite also might be true, with the proposed paper contributing new ideas and a different perspective to the topic. The review provides the background readings for the manuscript and may help the author to decide how to present the content to best meet the needs of particular readers.

The second purpose is to identify gaps in knowledge and where questions remain. Research studies and other types of projects should build on prior work and fill those gaps.

The third purpose is to determine how the proposed study or project will contribute new knowledge to nursing. How does the work contribute to the literature and answer existing questions? How does it reinforce what is already known? Answering these questions is important later in the writing process, when the author describes the research or project in the manuscript, because readers are interested in how the work expanded the existing knowledge base of the topic.

Although this chapter presents guidelines for conducting literature reviews when writing a manuscript, these same principles apply when reviewing the literature for papers for courses, a thesis, a dissertation, grants, and projects in which the nurse may be involved.

Literature Reviews for Papers for Courses

When writing the literature review for a term paper and other papers for courses, the author begins with identifying a topic (or the one assigned by the teacher), locates research and other types of articles on that topic using bibliographic databases, critiques and synthesizes the literature, and then writes the review. The keys to this process are understanding the purpose of the paper and pacing oneself to have adequate time to complete the review and write the necessary number of drafts of the paper.

Literature Reviews for Theses and Dissertations

For a thesis, which is a master's level research project, and a dissertation, which is a more extensive and original research study completed at the doctoral level, the same process is used for completing the literature review. The student begins with a topic, approved by the faculty advisor, and then locates, critiques, and synthesizes prior research, identifying how the study contributes new knowledge to nursing or confirms what is already known about the topic.

The literature review for a thesis and dissertation is comprehensive, revealing studies about the problem and related areas, and provides the rationale for conducting the research. The student needs to be thorough in identifying the relevant literature, use preset criteria for analyzing studies, and synthesize findings to reveal what is known about the problem and what needs to be examined further. Students defend the research proposal and completed thesis and dissertation under the scrutiny of the student's committee and other faculty, depending on the procedures established by the college and university. The literature review is a major part of this process, providing the background and rationale for conducting the study and demonstrating how the completed research adds new knowledge to nursing.

Literature Reviews for Grants and Projects

Nurses review and critique the literature as background for developing grants and projects. The literature review provides the rationale for the grant and project, indicating how they fulfill important needs. Depending on their purposes, the types of literature reviewed may include original research reports, descriptive articles, anecdotal reports, monographs, books, and even published case reports. The process of conducting and writing the literature review is similar to other types of papers.

Literature Reviews for Manuscripts

The literature review completed for a course assignment, thesis, dissertation, grant, and project may lead to the preparation of a manuscript and serve as the basis for writing its introduction and literature review section, depending on the format of the manuscript. For other manuscripts, though, the author begins with an idea and then searches the literature to learn what has already been published on the topic and to develop the background for the paper. Regardless of the beginning point for the literature review, the same process is used for identifying, critiquing, and synthesizing the literature.

There are differences, though, in how the literature is presented in a manuscript compared with these earlier papers. In a manuscript, there are restrictions in the number of pages, and the author needs to limit the summary of the literature to allow adequate pages for other sections of the paper. As such, the literature reviews in most manuscripts are short and focused, providing the background of the topic and rationale for the research or project described in the manuscript.

Format to Use

Each journal has its own format, which includes how the literature is reported. In many journals, the literature is integrated in the introduction. With this format, the introduction presents the topic of the paper, purpose of the research or project, and why the topic is important and uses the literature to present the background and rationale for the research or project.

In other journals, a section may be devoted to the literature review. With these papers, then, the topic and importance of it are discussed in the introduction, often using research and other types of articles as support. The literature then is presented in the next section of the paper.

Extent of Literature and Style of Presentation

The extent of literature presented and writing style used also differ across journals. For research manuscripts, the literature review is extensive and includes an analysis of prior studies and synthesis of the findings. Journals that publish research expect a comprehensive review of the literature (Heinrich, 2000).

But what about other journals? The research paper may be submitted to a clinical journal that also includes some reports of research. When writing for a journal that focuses more on clinical practice, the literature review will be less extensive. In many journals, the presentation of the literature emphasizes the practice implications of prior studies, and the author needs this information before writing the literature review.

It should be apparent why the earlier review of the journals, their goals, and their writing styles is important. This review gives the author a sense of the extent of literature to be presented in a particular journal and how that literature should be reported. In some journals, a more formal and academic style of writing is used to present the literature, whereas in other journals an informal style is used. An example of each style is presented in Display 5.1.

Literature: Current and Reported Accurately

Manuscripts submitted to refereed journals are peer reviewed before acceptance and, if published, are critically read by others. The literature cited in the paper should present the current state of the research on the topic and should be accurate. For a research paper, the author may have completed the litera-

DISPLAY 5.1   **Writing Styles for Literature Reviews**

FORMAL, ACADEMIC STYLE

Research in nursing related to consumer assessment of health care quality has focused predominantly on patient satisfaction with care, particularly nursing care in hospitals (Chang, 1997; Hinshaw & Atwood, 1992; Jacox, Bausell, & Mahrenholz, 1997; Minnick & Young, 1999) and outpatient care settings (Ketefian, Redman, Nash, & Bogue, 1997). Patient satisfaction is influenced by patients' expectations and how they define quality of care. Providers' perceptions of quality, however, may differ from patients' perceptions (Larrabee, 1995; Lynn & McMillan 1999; Lynn & Moore, 1997).[1]

INFORMAL STYLE

Many studies have been done in nursing on patient satisfaction with their nursing care in hospitals and outpatient clinics (Chang, 1997; Ketefian, Redman, Nash, & Bogue, 1997). We know from these studies that patients expect a certain level of nursing care, and these expectations influence their satisfaction with care. Nurses do not always know what elements of nursing care are important to patients—we need to learn more about this from our patients (Lynn & McMillan, 1999).

[1]From Oermann, M.H., & Templin, T. (2000). Important attributes of quality health care: Consumer perspectives. *Journal of Nursing Scholarship, 32,* 168. Reprinted with permission of Sigma Theta Tau.

ture review a year or more before beginning the manuscript; in these cases, the literature review probably will need to be updated. The author should cite the latest work published on the topic.

Accuracy is essential in interpreting and summarizing the literature as well as in citing the references. Errors in citing references in the text of papers and on the reference lists must be avoided because inaccurate citations give the impression of "sloppy scholarship" and may impede the retrieval of documents (Taylor, 1998).

REVIEW CLASSIFICATION

There are different ways of classifying the literature that might be reviewed for papers in nursing. One way of categorizing the literature is by empirical, theoretical, descriptive, anecdotal reports, and literature and integrative reviews. The literature also includes primary and secondary sources.

Empirical

The empirical literature includes reports of research published in journals and books as well as unpublished studies such as master's theses and doctoral dissertations. These are the original reports of the research. In writing research papers, the author focuses predominantly on empirical literature. Because the author has reviewed this literature as a basis for developing the research proposal and conducting the study, frequently only newly published articles need to be examined before beginning the manuscript.

Theoretical

Theoretical articles describe concepts, models, and theories in nursing and related fields. These articles are valuable for developing a conceptual framework for a research study.

Descriptive

Many articles in nursing journals do not describe research or theory but instead report on practices important to nurses regardless of their role. Articles on topics such as patient care, new clinical practices, trends in nursing, educational innovations, nursing management, and nursing issues are in this category of literature. These are important articles because they provide the background information for a manuscript and allow the author to assess what others have written about the topic.

Anecdotal Reports

Anecdotal reports are articles built around personal experiences rather than planned research on a topic. An article about the benefits of preceptors to new graduates based on comments by the graduates, preceptors' evaluations, and observations by others in the clinical setting is an example of an anecdotal report; the effects of using preceptors were not measured through research. Galvan (1999) cautions about using anecdotal reports as a source of information in literature reviews because they lack control.

Literature and Integrative Reviews

Some journals publish articles that are reviews of the literature. Literature reviews summarize what is known about a particular topic, and integrative reviews critique past research and draw overall conclusions from the body of literature (Beyea & Nicoll, 1998). Journals that publish review articles usually have high standards for these papers. Reviews are valuable to authors in writing for publication because they synthesize the current state of the literature, indicating for the author what is already known and gaps in knowledge.

Primary and Secondary Sources

Primary sources are original sources of information written by the person who developed the ideas. They are original because they are the first published accounts of the research, theory, and idea. For empirical research, the primary source is the paper written by the researcher who conducted the study. In primary sources, the reader finds detailed information about the research problem, methodology, results, and discussion written by the researchers themselves.

In the theoretical literature, the primary source is the theorist who developed the model, theory, or framework. For other types of literature, the primary source is the originator of the idea.

In secondary sources, the information is summarized and reported by someone other than the originator. Summaries of research, descriptions of clinical projects, and discussions of models and theories reported in articles, books, and other references by an author other than the original are secondary sources. The problem with using secondary sources is that the author has interpreted and summarized the writings of someone else. With secondary sources on research, sometimes only limited information is provided about the methodology and findings or the discussion may highlight only some of the important outcomes.

For secondary theoretical literature, authors may have misinterpreted the model, theory, or framework or allowed their own views to influence the discussion. For other literature, authors of secondary sources may omit vital details that would influence use of the ideas in practice and may be biased in the information reported and how it is presented in the paper.

In searching the literature for research purposes and for writing research papers, only primary literature should be used. Secondary sources should be included only if primary sources cannot be found or if the secondary source has a creative idea or unique organization not found in the primary source (Burns & Grove, 1999).

 ## DIFFERENCES IN LITERATURE REVIEWS FOR RESEARCH AND USE IN PRACTICE

Literature reviews for developing a research proposal and writing a research paper differ from those conducted when the goal is to locate background information about patient care, an issue faced in practice, a project being considered, and other topics not related to planning or reporting research.

Review for Research Purposes

Literature reviews for research purposes examine studies already completed on the research question and related topics to better understand the problem, identify gaps in the research, and provide a basis for conducting the study. These literature reviews are mainly of empirical literature. A literature review of this type informs the researcher of what has already been learned about the topic, which questions remain, and how the proposed research contributes to answering those questions (Martin, 1997).

While the study is being conducted, the researcher continues to periodically review the literature to keep current with other relevant studies. When the researcher then is ready to publish the findings of the study, a follow-up literature review may be needed, depending on how consistently the literature was reviewed up to this point.

The literature review presents prior research, not descriptions of practice nor anecdotal reports. Nonresearch articles, though, found in the literature review provide sources of information for the author to use in writing the introduction and the discussion section of the paper. They contribute to establishing the background of the problem, and they enable the author to make a case about why the study was indicated.

The other type of literature typically reviewed for research proposals and papers relates to theoretical literature, which describes concepts and theories to guide the research. A review of theoretical articles and books provides the background for developing the conceptual framework for the research study and for understanding the research results. Theories often enable the researcher to organize the literature around concepts in the theory and link together pieces of information and evidence from a study.

Quantitative Research

In quantitative studies, the literature review directs the development and implementation of the study (Burns & Grove, 1999). The literature is examined before beginning the study to identify the work already done on the topic and where further study is indicated. The background and significance of the study are developed from the review of the literature. Theoretical literature is used to construct the conceptual framework for the research. The methodology, including the design, sample, measurement, and data collection procedure, is based on previous research (Burns & Grove, 1999). The literature review also is used in analyzing the data and reporting the findings, so the current research builds on earlier studies.

In quantitative studies, the literature review is used in each phase of the research. Relevant literature may be cited throughout the research paper except for the results section. Generally, no references to the literature are included in the results section of the paper.

Qualitative Research

In qualitative research, however, the literature review varies according to the type of study. The role of the literature is different in a qualitative study, informing the results rather than shaping the discussion (Zaruba, Toma, & Stark, 1996). Burns and Grove (1999, p. 108) indicate that in phenomenological research, the literature is reviewed after the data are collected and analyzed to avoid influencing the thinking of the researcher and to help the researcher remain objective. For grounded theory studies, whereas some literature may be examined before the data are collected, to gain a perspective of prior work in the area, the literature is used predominantly to explain and extend the theory generated from the research.

Sandelowski (1998, p. 376) suggests that there is no one style for presenting qualitative research; researchers choose the "story" they will tell in the manuscript and how to tell it. For qualitative manuscripts, the style and format of the paper and how the literature is presented depend on the purposes of the research, methods used, and data.

Review for Use in Practice

Literature reviews also are done for application to clinical practice, teaching, and administration. By reviewing the literature, nurses gain an understanding of information on best practices for nursing, new approaches to patient care, and trends in nursing and health care that will guide their practice. Varied types of literature may be examined including descriptive articles, books, anecdotal reports, case reports, and empirical studies.

A comprehensive literature review that involves both a critique and synthesis of research provides a framework for developing evidence-based practices in nursing whether the focus is patient care, teaching, or administration. An integrative literature review summarizes past research and draws conclusions from the literature; this type of review is one way of documenting the scientific base of nursing practice (Beyea & Nicoll, 1998).

Similar to research reports, if the author reviewed the literature as a basis for developing a project, an innovation, or another endeavor, when ready to write the manuscript, the author often needs to update and expand the literature review. One literature review as a basis for developing new standards of practice, for instance, may not be sufficient for writing later about those standards and how they were used and evaluated in the clinical setting.

BEGINNING THE SEARCH

The author begins the literature review by identifying the topic of the paper. Whether the review is for a course, a thesis or dissertation, a research study, a project, or an idea to be developed into a manuscript, the author begins with a general topic and then narrows it down to one that can searched easily in a bibliographic database. For example, the author may plan to write a manuscript on a project to improve the satisfaction of patients with their care in the clinic. The topic "consumer satisfaction" is too broad for reviewing the literature; there are nearly 23,000 publications indexed in the MEDLINE® (Medical Literature, Analysis, and Retrieval System Online) database alone on this topic. Narrowing the topic to patient satisfaction with nursing care in ambulatory settings produces a more manageable literature review with about 50 citations.

Bibliographic Databases

The author then searches the literature. This had been done earlier by looking up references in the card catalog and in the annual indexes of the periodical literature, which were only in print format. This information is now compiled in electronic databases, which can be accessed using the Internet or may be provided on a local area network or in the library. These databases are searched electronically, making them fast and easy to use. Each publication in the database is reviewed, a record is produced that describes the publication and its characteristics, and then the content is indexed. This allows the user to search the database for specific content areas and other information.

Bibliographic databases, such as MEDLINE, include the citations and the related indexing information. They help the author find information resources (Allen, 1999). Some databases, however, go a step further and provide the complete indexed document. These are called full-text databases because they link to the complete document rather than only providing information about it.

Many libraries now have electronic databases with records for references held by the library or by a group of libraries. Searching these databases is similar to looking up references using the card catalog. The database can be searched by key word, author, title, subject heading, journal title, and call number. Some of the library on-line catalogs may be accessed using the Internet, allowing them to be searched from home and other settings in addition to the library.

Bibliographic Databases for Nursing Literature

There are varied bibliographic databases for conducting literature searches in nursing. For literature reviews related to nursing practice, the two most useful databases are MEDLINE and the Cumulative Index to Nursing and Allied Health Literature (CINAHL®); both index journal articles. CINAHL also indexes other types of information resources valuable to nurses in writing for publication. When the paper extends beyond nursing journals, other bibliographic databases—such as PsychINFO for literature on psychology and related subject areas—may be used for the search. In addition, many authors use the library catalog, which may be on line, to locate books and other types of resources. Selecting the database to search is discussed later in the chapter.

Because many authors use personal computers for writing their manuscripts at home and in settings convenient for them, on-line databases provide easy access to nursing literature when the author is ready to complete a literature review or needs to update the review. With Internet access, some of the databases can be searched from home for no charge, such as MEDLINE, or by subscription.

MEDLINE

The National Library of Medicine (NLM) provides a wide variety of resources related to the biomedical and health sciences. These resources include the following: searchable databases and databanks, bibliographic citations, full text (when available), archival collections, and images. Links to the many resources of the NLM can be found at *http://www.nlm.nih.gov*. The Library's catalog of books, journals, audiovisuals, and access points to other medical research tools can be reached through LOCATORplus. Consumers can find health information on line through MEDLINEplus at *http://www.nlm.nih.gov/ medlineplus*.

There are varied databases that can be searched for literature reviews. A list of these databases with links is available at *http://www.nlm.nih.gov/ databases/databases.html*. MEDLINE, one of these databases, is an on-line bibliographic database of literature in medicine, nursing, dentistry, veterinary medicine, the health care system, and preclinical sciences. MEDLINE also covers life sciences, including some aspects of biology, environmental science, marine biology, plant and animal science, biophysics, and chemistry (NLM, 2000a).

Citations in MEDLINE are from more than 4,000 biomedical journals worldwide, published mainly in English. MEDLINE contains over 11 million references to journal articles, including many from nursing journals. The database is updated weekly (NLM, 2000a).

MEDLINE is available on the Internet through the NLM home page at *http://www.nlm.nih.gov*. The link from the NLM home page is to two Web-based services, PubMed® and Internet Grateful Med. Both of these enable the author to begin a MEDLINE search. The author also can go directly to these sites. MEDLINE can be searched for free, and no registration is required. Access to various MEDLINE services often is available from medical libraries and many public libraries.

MEDLINE was the first on-line database that indexed journal articles, beginning in 1966. As such, the database includes articles published since that date; earlier works are available through OLDMEDLINE, which can be accessed through PubMed and Internet Grateful Med.

MEDLINE is easy to search. Articles are indexed using medical subject headings (MeSH®), which is the NLM system to index articles and to catalog books. MEDLINE can be searched using MeSH or by author name, title word, text word, journal name, phrase, or any combination of these (NLM, 2000b). A search produces a list of citations to journal articles. These citations include the author, title, source of the article, and abstract if available. Citations found during the search can be saved on a clipboard, and articles of interest may be ordered, for a fee, through Loansome Doc.

CINAHL

The CINAHL is a comprehensive database of nursing literature. It also covers literature in allied health disciplines and other subjects such as biomedicine, alternative medicine, and consumer health. The index is available in print format and on line.

In 1961, the first edition of CINAHL was published, indexing the literature from 1956 to 1960 from 16 journals. Now articles from more than 1,200 journals are indexed in CINAHL. Of these journals, more than 400 are nursing journals (CINAHL, 2000). The electronic database includes indexing since 1982, as well as nursing dissertations, educational software, audiovisuals, abstracts from more than 800 journals, selected full-text articles, and critical paths. Journals covered in CINAHL can be searched alphabetically or by subject.

Full text is included for selected state nursing journals, standards of practice, government publications, research instruments, legal cases, drug information, and patient education materials. Researchers can review a list of research instruments in the CINAHL database.

In 1994, CINAHL initiated the citation index. The citations in the database can be used to track the development of ideas in nursing and work of particular authors. The index also can be used to follow the progress of research in nursing and how research findings have been used in clinical practice and other areas of nursing.

Material is indexed according to the CINAHL Subject Heading List specifically designed for nursing and allied health literature. The structure is based on MeSH but includes added terms and phrases that are tailored to meet the needs of nursing and allied health professionals.

CINAHL also has specialty databases that allow the author to retrieve current literature in a specialty area; these often are helpful when beginning a literature review. The specialty databases are in advanced nursing practice, case management, critical care, emergency care, gerontology, home health, obstetrics, oncology, and perioperative care (CINAHL, 2000).

The CINAHL database is available at medical libraries and libraries with health information; employees and students more than likely can access the database for no charge. Personal subscriptions to CINAHL are available on CD-ROM or on line through one of the CINAHL vendors or CINAHLdirect® on-line service. There is a subscription fee. With a subscription, CINAHL can be accessed at all times, similar to MEDLINE. Authors are able to obtain copies of the journal articles both on line and by mail or fax through CINAHLexpress. Selected articles stored as PDF files are available for immediate downloading. These services make it easy to complete literature reviews at times convenient for the author.

International Nursing Index

The International Nursing Index (INI) is another index available for conducting literature reviews in nursing. It is based on the nursing journals indexed in MEDLINE and also includes doctoral dissertations in nursing. The INI is published in cooperation with the NLM and presents the indexing from MEDLINE for over 300 nursing journals.

Other Bibliographic Databases

For many manuscripts, the author needs to review the literature in areas other than nursing. It is worth the time before beginning the paper to conduct a thorough search of the literature using multiple databases if appropriate. This provides the author with a broad view of what has already been published on the topic, not only the work done in nursing. Selecting other databases to review depends on the topic of the manuscript.

A brief description of selected other databases is found in Table 5.1. This list is not exhaustive but provides an example of the wealth of databases that might be used for reviewing the literature.

Database Structure

Each publication in a bibliographic database has a single record with fields that contain specific information describing the publication. For instance, the record for a book would include the author's name, title of the book, edition, publisher, and date. Allen (1999) refers to this information as descriptive data. There also are fields in the record to indicate the main subject or subjects covered in the book; a cataloger assigns subject headings and a call number after reviewing the content in the book (Allen, 1999). The subject headings and number assigned are based on the classification system used by the library.

Each article in a bibliographic database is indexed similarly. It has a single record with specific information about that article. The record has fields, which include information such as the author's name, title of the article, journal in which published, publication date and information, and terms or phrases that describe the content of the article. These terms or phrases are important in searching the literature, although sometimes the writer may begin by searching for particular authors who have done similar work.

TABLE 5.1

Selected Bibliographic Databases

Database	Subject Area
BioSciences Citation Index (ISI Citation Database)	Multidisciplinary database of life science journals
CINAHL	Nursing and allied health literature
Clinical Medicine Citation Index (ISI Citation Database)	Multidisciplinary database covering publications in clinical research
Dissertation Abstracts	Abstracts of dissertations in all subjects accepted at U.S. institutions; access to abstracts online through Dissertation Abstracts Online
EMBASE	On-line counterpart to *Excerpta Medica* covering biomedical literature and, notably, drug research and information
ERIC	Database contains more than 1 million abstracts of documents and articles in field of education (including research and practice)
HEALTHSTAR	On-line database covering literature on health care administration, economics, planning, and policy; health services research; and health care technology assessment
MEDLINE	Medicine, nursing, dentistry, veterinary medicine, the health care system, and preclinical sciences
National Library of Medicine Databases	MEDLINE and many other on-line databases such as BIOETHICSLINE on ethical, legal, and public policy issues of health care; CANCERLIT, which provides access to cancer information; AIDSLINE, AIDSDRUGS, and AIDSTRIALS databases covering HIV/AIDS literature and research; and HISTLINE database on the history of medicine and related subjects
RNdex™	Citations to articles from more than 150 nursing and case management journals; selected citations from related health care and critical care medicine journals, supplement nursing journals
Psychological Abstracts	Psychology, psychological disorders, and related fields; on-line counterpart is PsycINFO
Science Citation Index (ISI Citation Database)	Multidisciplinary database of science journal literature; nearly 6,000 journals indexed

(continued)

TABLE 5.1	
Selected Bibliographic Databases (Continued)	
Database	**Subject Area**
Wilson Social Sciences Abstracts	Abstracting and indexing of more than 400 journals in areas of anthropology, criminology, economics, law, geography, policy studies, psychology, sociology, social work, and urban studies
Social Sciences Citation Index (ISI Citation Database)	Multidisciplinary database covering journal literature of social sciences
Social Work Abstracts Plus	Database covering more than 450 journals related to social work and human services including theory and practice, areas of service, social issues, and social problems
Sociological Abstracts	Access to theoretical and applied sociology, social science, and policy science journal citations and abstracts; chapter, book, and association paper abstracts; book, film, and software review citations

Terms for Indexing

The NLM uses MeSH, which is a controlled vocabulary thesaurus. A thesaurus is a carefully constructed set of terms often connected by links that show the relationship between terms. A thesaurus also is referred to as a "classification structure" or an "ordering system" (NLM, 2000b). MeSH is used for MED-LINE indexing and other databases produced by the NLM.

MeSH consists of a set of terms or subject headings that are arranged in both an alphabetical and a hierarchical structure (NLM, 2000b). It uses a tree structure whereby terms are grouped under broad headings, which then have more specific subject headings under them. At the most general level of the hierarchical structure are broad headings such as "education," and at narrower levels are more specific headings such as "baccalaureate nursing education." Display 5.2 provides an example of the MeSH subject headings and levels for the topic "baccalaureate nursing education."

CINAHL has its own controlled vocabulary thesaurus based on MeSH but with additional terms for nursing and allied health literature (Allen, 1998). A major advantage of using CINAHL is that the search terms are intended for the nursing literature. For example, if the author is preparing a paper describing a nursing model or theory, there is a major heading on nursing theory, with many different models and theories listed by both the author's last name and formal name of the model or theory. To learn how theories are used in a research study, the main subject heading would pertain to the research topic

DISPLAY 5.2	**Example of MeSH Subject Headings**

Anthropology, education, sociology, and social phenomena category
  Education
    Education, professional
      Education, nursing
        Education, nursing, associate
        Education, nursing, baccalaureate
        Education, nursing, continuing
        Education, nursing, diploma program
        Education, nursing, graduate
        Education, nursing, research

such as effectiveness of nursing interventions for chronic pain. The theories that guided the research, though, such as Orem's self-care theory or quality of life, would be indexed as minor headings. By expanding the search beyond the major subject headings, the search would retrieve studies using these theories as their frameworks. The search in MEDLINE would be less precise because there is only a general heading on nursing models.

As another example, if the author is writing a paper on a new staffing pattern for maternity nursing, CINAHL contains a subject heading in for obstetric nursing and other headings such as hospital units, nursing care, alternative birth centers, and primary nursing. The many subheadings for obstetric nursing might be searched, depending on the focus of the paper (eg, administration, economics, manpower, organizations, and trends).

Table 5.2 compares the major terms for an article indexed in MEDLINE and the same article in CINAHL. The terms in CINAHL are more specific to the nursing literature.

How Terms are Selected

When articles are indexed in a database, an indexer decides what terms or phrases best represent the content in the article. These terms, though, are not decided individually by each indexer but instead are selected from the database thesaurus (Allen, 1999). The task of the indexer is to choose subject headings from the thesaurus that best represent the article. This ensures that all articles on a particular subject are indexed in the same way, which is essential when searching for that information.

Key Words

The indexed terms often are called key words in the author guidelines for journals. The guidelines often ask authors to submit a short list of key words with

TABLE 5.2
Sample Comparison of Subject Indexing in MEDLINE and CINAHL

Author: McGregor RJ
Title: A Precepted Experience for Senior Students
Source: Nurse Educator 1999 May–June, 24(3):13–16

MEDLINE Terms	CINAHL Subject Headings
Curriculum	Education, nursing, baccalaureate
Decision making	Faculty role
Education, nursing, baccalaureate/ organization & administration	Faculty, nursing
	Interinstitutional relations
Human	Mentorship
Preceptorship	Preceptorship
Program evaluation	Student placement
Students, nursing	Students, nursing, baccalaureate
	Teaching methods, clinical

the manuscript when it is submitted. These words then are used for indexing the paper if it is accepted. To identify key words, go to the thesaurus of the database in which the journal is indexed and select key words that best describe the content. The databases usually are listed in the journal on the masthead or table of contents page. If unsure of where the journal is indexed, use MeSH terms or CINAHL subject headings.

Selecting the Database

After choosing the topic and narrowing it down, the next step is to select the most appropriate database for the search. For most clinical topics in nursing, the author uses the library catalog and both CINAHL and MEDLINE databases. Burnham and Shearer (1993) conducted a study to determine which of three databases, CINAHL, MEDLINE, and EMBASE (on-line Excerpta Medica), should be accessed when researching nursing topics. From their findings, they suggest searching both CINAHL and MEDLINE to retrieve information on a clinical topic. Searches on nonclinical topics often extend beyond these into other relevant databases, such as those listed in Table 5.1. If unsure of which databases to use, the author should consult with a librarian or should review potential databases and types of articles indexed in them.

Deciding on which databases to search is important for the author because critical articles may be missed in the search. Even though on-line resources are easy to access and convenient to use, a comprehensive search also may involve a review of books and other sources of information.

 ## SEARCH STRATEGIES

Once the databases are selected, it is wise to become familiar with how they are organized. Read through some records of articles indexed in them to gain a perspective of the fields and information provided. Many of the databases offer differ views of each record. For instance, one view may include the citation and abstract only, whereas another view adds the terms (eg, MeSH terms or CINAHL subject headings) and other indexing information.

Before beginning the search:

- Become familiar with the database and the literature indexed in it.
- Learn how the database is organized and how to use it for a search.
- Review sample records and different views of each record.
- Locate the thesaurus and look up the terms that might be used for the search.
- Review search strategies and tips included with information about the database.
- Learn how to broaden the search (eg, by using *or*), narrow the search (eg, by using *and*), exclude terms in a search (eg, by using *not*), and other ways of making the search more precise.
- Learn how to save searches while in progress and at their completion.
- Determine how to order documents if available.

Selecting Search Terms

After selecting an appropriate database, do a quick search to determine how much literature has been published on the topic. Begin by looking up in the thesaurus of the database the terms to use for the search. This preliminary search helps the author determine how to restate the terms if needed before beginning the actual search.

The initial search may reveal that the terms chosen are too broad and need to be more specific to produce more manageable results. If the author is planning on writing a manuscript on using videotapes for teaching patients with asthma, searching in PubMed by using "patient education" yields 30,000 citations. The term "asthma" results in 60,000 citations. The author needs to choose more specific terms from the thesaurus to best describe the topic and retrieve relevant articles or modify the search using other techniques. At the other extreme, the terms initially selected for the search may be too specific, thereby excluding some of the relevant literature.

Combining Search Terms

Searches can be modified by choosing other terms to search; by manipulating the fields such as limiting publication dates, looking for selected authors, or restricting the search to certain journals; and by using the Boolean connectors *and, or,* and *not.* These connectors indicate how the computer should combine the search terms and treat them in relation to one another. *And* indicates that both of the terms it connects must be found in the citation or abstract; *or* means that the citations must contain at least one of the selected terms; and *not* means to exclude citations with the selected term (NLM, 2000b).

In the example on a search of the literature on videotapes for teaching patients with asthma, by including *and* between "patient education" *and* "asthma," the list is reduced to approximately 1,000 references, but this still is too many to be manageable. Limiting the search to English language produces about 900 citations. Even restricting these to the last 5 years yields nearly 500 citations. About 190 articles were published in the current year alone; depending on the purpose of the paper and literature review, the author might decide to review these citations for the most relevant ones. This literature would provide background information on educating patients with asthma though not necessarily by using videotapes as the instructional method.

The author may decide to add "videotapes" to the search; a look in the MeSH browser reveals that "videotape recordings" is the term for searching, not videotapes. This revision in the search yields nine citations, which are too few for the complete search but represent citations that should be reviewed by the author.

Searching for "asthma" and "videotape recordings" results in 20 citations, all of which should be reviewed. Some of the references, though, pertain to use of videotape for noninstructional purposes, and the author can exclude these quickly by reading the abstract of the article.

Modifying the search to "patient education" and "videotape recordings" results in about 250 citations. Limiting the publication date to the last 5 years, though, produces approximately 80 citations, a more manageable number. Although these articles do not focus on videotapes for teaching patients with asthma, they provide background information on how videotapes have been used for educating patients with other health problems and in varied settings. For example, there are articles on informational videotapes for patients in the emergency department, comparing the effectiveness of video and print materials for educating clinic patients with sleep disorders, and using videotape instruction for other groups of patients. This literature would contribute to a better understanding of what is known about educating patients by videotape instruction and as such should be reviewed by the author.

This is a good example of how different terms might be combined to retrieve the best citations for the paper and a manageable number without omitting important publications. The author should allow time to experiment with terms and phrases until the search produces the type of literature needed for preparing the paper.

Searching Relevant Databases

With the search strategy planned, the author is ready to begin the search in all relevant databases. The search of the database used to refine the search terms should be done first, then the author should move to other databases if appropriate. The author should check the thesaurus of each database because different terms and phrases may be used. The search also includes books and other resources that might contribute to the background of the manuscript.

When the author finds a relevant citation, some databases allow for searching related articles. This feature produces a list of citations to articles that are indexed with the same terms or similar ones.

Reviewing the Literature: How Far Back?

The literature should be reviewed starting with the most recent references and working backward. When restricting the publication dates to the most recent, which usually is done, the author should be alert to landmark or classic studies that might have been published earlier.

Determining how far back to review the literature depends on the topic. Reviewing literature published in the last 5 years usually is sufficient for most papers. If there are limited publications in this time frame, then the author can continue to work backward, asking why there are few recent publications. The problem may lie with the search terms, or it may suggest to the author that trends in nursing should be considered in the paper. Some areas of nursing practice, such as technology, are changing so rapidly that articles published a few years earlier are outdated.

Reviewing Reference Lists

As the citations of articles, books, and other resources are retrieved, the author may decide to extend the search using alternate terms or even searching different databases. One other technique is to review the reference lists of the articles, chapters, and books to identify other citations that might have been missed. The classic references sometimes are found there. The author also may find citations to journals not in the databases used for the original search or may identify other subject headings that might extend the search.

CINAHL includes the reference lists with articles in its database. This makes it easy for authors to extend their searches from one citation to others.

Completing the Search

A word of caution: there comes a point at which the author must decide to complete the search and begin writing the manuscript. Otherwise, the author may delay writing and use valuable time to locate a few more references not even needed for preparation of the paper.

Keeping Records

The following are guidelines for recording the results of literature searches. The list is not exhaustive but includes some strategies to manage the searches and keep track of records reviewed.

- Keep a record of (1) each database searched, (2) terms used for the search, (3) years searched, (4) limitations placed on the search such as English language publications only, and (5) resulting citations. Mark the date the search was completed. This record should be kept for writing the current paper and for subsequent searches on the same topic.

- Record the search terms on a file card (eg, 3 × 5 inch index card) or in a computer file, including terms originally chosen by the author and those from the thesaurus of the database. Include any synonyms for the original terms and note which terms are not effective so that this information is available for later searches.

- Record explicitly how search terms were combined and the citations produced from each combination.

- Note the dates of any changes in search terms so that there is a running record of the progression of the search.

- If related records were searched, make a note of how these were accessed and resulting citations.

- Note citations identified from reference lists of articles, chapters, and books, including the original reference.

- Keep a list of all citations from each search and organize these to avoid reviewing the same reference more than once. With on-line searching, the list of citations can be printed.

- Record articles, chapters, books, and other materials that will not be used for the paper. If another search is done, this will avoid rechecking the same publication.

- Keep a record of documents ordered.
- Make a copy of publications that will be used in preparing the paper. This enables the author to have the material on hand when beginning to write.
- Record all information about a reference that might be needed because reference formats differ across journals. This avoids having to recheck a reference when a manuscript is submitted to a different journal, which may use a different format from the journal originally planned. Never rely on memory when it comes to references.

 ## MANAGING REFERENCES

Considering the numerous references retrieved in a search, authors need efficient ways of managing these references and retrieving them for research, writing, and other projects. Frequently, a literature search done for one purpose may be expanded for subsequent papers and projects. Along the same line, a review completed for a research study provides the basis for manuscripts written later. It is important to have a system for keeping track of references for the current project and for use in the future.

Developing Own System

For limited searches of the literature, it is possible to record the bibliographic information and even a brief summary of the content on 3 × 5 inch cards, but this is not an efficient way to keep track of references for most literature reviews. Cards get misplaced and can be stored only in one place at a time, limiting access to them. Keeping reference information in computer files with bibliographic software is more efficient and promotes easy access to the references. Authors can develop their own computerized bibliographic files to store information about references or can use commercial bibliographic management software.

Using Bibliographic Management Software

Instead of creating one's own bibliographic database, authors can purchase bibliographic management software, such as, EndNote, Reference Manager, and ProCite (ISI Research Soft, 2000). These software programs allow authors to search on-line bibliographic databases, store thousands of records, organize references in a database, create bibliographies automatically, and share references with others. They also enable authors to format manuscripts—complete with in-text citations—and bibliographies from within Microsoft Word and WordPerfect for more than 500 bibliographic styles for a variety of journals. If the author decides later to submit the manuscript to another publication, which uses a different reference style, the software reformats the in-text citations and bibliography. This avoids retyping them.

If interested in purchasing bibliographic management software, choose one that is versatile and easy to use. Try out the demonstration versions before purchasing.

 ## ANALYSIS OF THE LITERATURE

The author has searched the literature and is now ready to read and analyze the materials. In this phase of the literature review, the author organizes the publications into content areas, develops a format for recording comments, and then analyzes each publication.

Organizing Publications

Initially, the author should scan the materials to gain an overview of each publication and its content. This prereading enables the author to develop a perspective of the literature as a whole before reading separate and sometimes narrow reports (Galvan, 1999).

Then, the author groups the articles and other materials by topics or content areas that fit together. Although the publications usually are organized by topics, they also might be grouped chronologically or by research design and findings. The decision about how to organize them depends on the purpose of the paper and content area. Organizing them into categories facilitates the literature review because then all of the articles and other materials about one topic are read at a time. This helps the author gain an understanding of the content and what has already been published about it and to manage an extensive literature review. Reading the materials in categories also is valuable when writing the draft because the author has grouped the literature that might be used to present each content area.

As the articles and other documents are grouped into topics, the author should attempt to identify more specific content areas, subtopics, that in turn help to organize the literature within each topic. For instance, in a literature review on assisted dying and nursing practice, Schwarz (1999) groups the literature into these topics: (1) concept of assisted dying, (2) views of expert nurse clinicians on nurses' roles in assisted dying, (3) implications of the American Nurses Association position statements, and (4) research studies on nurse-assisted dying. The literature associated with the first topic then was grouped into subtopics and reviewed beginning with the concept of "assistance in dying" and then progressing to public perceptions of assisted dying; nurse participation in assisted dying; and social, political, and legal aspects of assistance in dying (Schwarz, 1999).

Articles can be placed in file folders of specific content areas with accompanying notes stored with them or they can be highlighted. Self-adhesive, color-coded flags can be used to note important comments from the publications that are critical to the literature review or might be cited in the paper, to keep track of different research methods and subjects, to identify trends in findings of studies or the development of ideas, and to highlight other points. If using a computer for note taking, these, too, can be color coded with word-processing software to keep track of ideas during the literature review.

For Internet and electronic resources, a similar system should be set up for keeping track of their review. This system should include documenting how the Internet search was conducted, the material accessed at the Web site including the author's name and title of the document, the name of the Web site and its URL, and the date accessed. This information is needed for the reference list of the paper should the site be included in it.

Format for Recording Comments

Before reviewing the publications and other resources, decide how comments will be recorded. Whether they are written on note cards or copies of the publications, or entered into the computer, a consistent system should be used when making notations about the publications. This facilitates writing the manuscript and saves the author time later. When reading research articles, consistency in note taking is helpful in examining patterns across studies and later in synthesizing findings. Care should be taken when recording quotations so that they are accurate; the page number should be noted, which will avoid having to return to the reference at the writing stage.

Figures 5-1 to 5-4 provide sample formats for recording comments about different types of literature reviewed. Regardless of the format, the key is to develop a consistent method of documenting comments so useful later when writing the paper.

Guidelines for Analyzing Literature

For some papers, the author's intent in reviewing the literature is to learn what has already been on the published on the topic to decide whether to proceed with the manuscript. Once this is determined, then authors need to critically examine each publication before using it as a basis for their own research and writing. Not every document retrieved from a literature review may be used for preparing a manuscript. Some papers are not used because of poor quality; other times, the content is not relevant to the paper.

The questions in Display 5.3 are useful for analyzing nursing literature. These are general questions to guide the critique of articles and other documents for deciding whether to include them in a literature review, assessing their

REFERENCE INFORMATION*

Article:

Authors' last name and first name†, middle initial(s) _____

Title of article _____

Journal name, volume, issue, and page numbers _____

Year of publication _____

Book:

Chapter authors' last and first names, initial(s) (if cited) _____

Title of chapter and page numbers (if cited) _____

Book authors'/editors' last and first names, initial(s) _____

Title of book and subtitle if any _____

Volume number and title if more than 1 volume; edition number
(other than 1st edition) _____

Place of publication, name of publisher, year of publication _____

Internet Materials:

Authors' last and first names†, middle initial(s) _____

Title of document _____

Name of web site _____

URL _____

Date accessed _____

Figure 5-1. Format for notes about publications: Non-research. *(continues).*

Notes

1. What is the main point of this publication?

2. What are the major content areas included in it?

3. What background information will it contribute to the paper?

4. How might the publication be used for writing the paper?

5. What are strengths of the publication? Weaknesses?

6. Other comments:

*Record complete citation. If using bibliographic management software or have copy of reference, record enough information to match notes with reference.

†Some reference formats require first name of lead author.

Figure 5-1. (Continued).

strengths and weaknesses, and planning how they might be incorporated as background for a paper.

Research reports need to be critically evaluated to decide if the study can be used as a basis for the author's own research and to assess the implications of the findings for nursing practice (Fosbinder & Loveridge, 1996). Studies have strengths and flaws, which should be recognized by the researcher. Problems may exist in how the study was conceptualized and its rationale. There may be issues with the design: its methods, how variables were measured, the instruments used, procedures, and data analysis. The study might have been well designed, but a small sample size limits generalizing the findings to other groups and settings. There may problems with the statistical analysis or how themes were identified and labeled in qualitative studies. Display 5-4 provides a guide for critiquing the research literature in nursing.

SYNTHESIZING THE LITERATURE

From this critique of individual articles and other documents, the author develops a view of the literature as a whole and an understanding of what is known about the topic and what still needs to be learned. Synthesis gives the author a sense of how studies and other types of projects relate to one another and a perspective of how the author's own topic relates to prior work. Syn-

REFERENCE INFORMATION*

Article:

Authors' last and first names†, middle initial(s) _____

Title of article _____

Journal name, volume, issue, and page numbers _____

Year of publication _____

Purpose/ Research questions	
Design	
Sample (and size)	
Instruments (validity and reliability)	
Findings	
Comments	

* Record complete citation. If using bibliographic management software or have a copy of the reference, record enough information to match notes with reference.
†Some reference formats require first name of lead author.

Figure 5-2. Format for notes about research publications: Quantitative.

Author(s)/Year	Purpose/ Research questions	Design	Sample (and size)	Instruments (validity and reliability)	Findings	Comments

Note: Add column for treatment if relevant

Figure 5-3. Format for summarizing research articles.

REFERENCE INFORMATION*

Article:

Authors' last and first names†, middle initial(s) _____

Title of article _____

Journal name, volume, issue, and page numbers _____

Year of publication _____

Type of qualitative study	
Purpose	
Methods	
Sample	
Findings	
Comments	

* Record complete citation. If using bibliographic management software or have a copy of the reference, record enough information to match notes with reference.
†Some reference formats require first name of lead author.

Figure 5-4. Format for notes about research publications: Qualitative.

DISPLAY 5.3	Guide for Analyzing Nursing Literature

- What is the purpose of the article or other type of document, and is it consistent with the author's goals for writing the paper?
- What topics and subtopics are addressed in the article, and are these similar to the content planned for the author's own paper?
- Does the introduction state the problem, issue, and need, and its significance? Can similarities be drawn between these and the author's own work to be discussed in the paper? If not, how will the article be used in the preparation of the paper?
- Is there a clear and coherent rationale for why the article was written? Why it is important?
- If the article describes nursing practice, a project, or an innovation, is it comprehensive, providing readers with information essential to using the content in their own settings?
- If the article suggests a change in practice, is there evidence provided for this change?
- Is the literature review in the article accurate and up-to-date? Are primary sources used?
- Does the literature support the discussion and establish the background?
- Does the article make it clear how it fills gaps in the literature? Is this accurate?
- Does the article make significant contributions to the nursing field? Why or why not? What is the relationship between these contributions and the author's goals for writing another paper?
- What concepts, models, and theories are described in the article, and are they relevant to the author's paper? How can these be used to develop the paper?
- Are key terms defined similarly?
- Does the article provide solutions to the problem, issue, or need identified in the introduction? Are these solutions applicable to the author's own work?
- If the article evaluated the effectiveness of an intervention, was the methodology sound? Was it described sufficiently to be replicated?
- What is unique about the problem, issue, need, intervention, subjects, setting, and resources described in the article? Are these relevant to the author's own situation? Why or why not?
- What are strengths and weaknesses of the article? How can they be used in preparing the author's own paper?

thesizing the research literature is critical because it allows the author to identify relationships among studies, gaps in the research, and where further study is needed before using the findings in practice.

In developing evidence-based practice, the synthesis of related research provides the evidence to support a change in practice or indicates that further study is needed. Rosswurm and Larrabee (1999, p. 320) emphasize the importance of synthesizing the research literature as the basis for determining whether changes are indicated in nursing practice. If the synthesis provides enough evidence to support a change in practice, with minimal risks, then nurses can proceed with the change.

DISPLAY 5.4	Guide for Analyzing Research Literature in Nursing

✔ Title
  Does it describe the study? Is it informative?
✔ Abstract
  Does it emphasize the study's purpose, method, major findings, and conclusions?
  Is this a quantitative or qualitative study?
✔ Introduction
  Does it state the problem and its significance to nursing?
  Does the introduction provide the background and rationale for the study?
  What is the purpose of the study, and is it clear?
  If a conceptual framework is presented, does it relate to the purpose and describe the
    concepts underlying the study and their relationships?
✔ Literature review
  Is the literature critically reviewed?
  Are strengths and weaknesses of earlier studies presented?
  Does the review support the rationale for conducting the study as reported in the article?
  Is the literature review up-to-date?
  Are important studies included in it?
  Are primary sources used?
✔ Research questions or hypotheses
  Are the research questions or hypotheses clear, specific, and stated appropriately?
  Are variables defined if appropriate?
✔ Design
  Is the design consistent with the problem?
  What type of design is used?
  What are strengths and weaknesses of the design?
✔ Sample
  Is the sampling procedure described?
  What criteria were used to select the sample?
  Is the sample size adequate?
  Is the sample representative, and how will this affect generalizing the findings?
✔ Instruments
  Are the instruments described, and are they appropriate?
  Are they valid and reliable?
✔ Data collection procedure
  Is the procedure clearly described?
  Are methods for collecting qualitative data appropriate for the type of study?

(continued)

Now that each publication has been reviewed and analyzed, the author's task is to integrate these and present a summary in the manuscript. First, the author returns to the original purpose of completing the literature review. Was the goal to develop the background for a research study, answer questions about clinical practice, move toward evidence-based practice, develop new projects, or make

DISPLAY
5.4   **Guide for Analyzing Research Literature in Nursing** *(Continued)*

✔ Findings
   Are the findings interpreted correctly including any statistical analyses?
   Are the statistics used to analyze the data appropriate?
   Are the findings presented clearly and in relation to the study questions or hypotheses?
   Are the findings presented logically?
   Are any tables and figures easy to read, and do they support the text?
✔ Discussion
   Are the conclusions based on the study results?
   Is the discussion related to the literature, and does it include how the study builds on
     earlier research?
   Are the limitations identified, and could they have been resolved?
   Can the findings be generalized and if so, to what populations?
✔ Strengths and weaknesses
   Overall, what are the study's major strengths and weaknesses?

other decisions? Was the literature review conducted for a paper in a course, thesis, dissertation, grant, or project in which the nurse may be involved? Was the purpose of the literature review to decide whether to write the manuscript, and if so, how should it be developed to fill gaps in the literature? The synthesis should meet these original goals for reviewing the literature.

Second, for each topic and subtopic, the author should identify similarities and common points of view in the publications. For research reports, the author should note when findings are consistent across studies. When findings are different, the author should propose explanations for these differences (Galvan, 1999). For instance, were the studies done at varied points in time? Were there differences in methodologies and subjects that might account for the discrepancies in findings? Were different instruments used, or were there variations in statistical analyses that might account for the lack of consistency in the results?

Third, the author should recognize gaps in the literature. In writing the paper, the author makes a case how the paper fills these gaps and contributes new knowledge to nursing.

 WRITING THE LITERATURE REVIEW

The first step in writing the literature review is to consider the audience of the journal to which the manuscript will be submitted. If writing the literature review for a research journal, it should be comprehensive, each research study should be critiqued as described earlier, and research findings should be synthesized, noting where further study is indicated. In the review, authors should justify their study by pointing out how it

1. Closes a gap in the literature
2. Tests an important aspect of current theory
3. Replicates an important study
4. Extends earlier work using a different sample or improved methods and procedures
5. Resolves conflicts in the literature (Galvan, 1999, pp. 65–66).

For other journals, the literature review will not have the same depth, nor will readers expect this same level of critique as in a research journal. Often, the literature is used to present the topic and why it is important for readers. The literature may be integrated throughout the paper rather than discussed in a separate section. Again, the importance of identifying possible journals before writing the paper is apparent when deciding how to present the literature review.

Introductory Statement

The literature review should begin an introductory statement about what literature will be presented and why it is important to the problem or purpose of the paper. This introductory statement should not be too broad.

In the following example, the first introductory statement to the literature review is too broad; it does not tell the reader what types of literature will be discussed. The methods for assessing critical thinking could be standardized tests, strategies used in classroom instruction, or methods for evaluating critical thinking in clinical practice. The revised statement indicates more specifically that the literature reviewed is on methods for assessing the critical thinking of nursing students in clinical practice.

Broad:

Critical thinking is an important competency needed by nursing students. Varied methods can be used for assessing critical thinking.

Specific:

Five methods of assessing nursing students' critical thinking skills within the context of clinical practice are (1) observation of students in practice, (2) Socratic questions, (3) conferences, (4) problem-solving strategies, and (5) written assignments. The literature is reviewed on each of these methods.

Important Studies

In writing the literature review, the author should highlight important studies and describe why they are significant. Classic studies should be noted and some discussion provided as to how they contributed to nursing. These papers frequently are pivotal works in the development of the topic and can be used in the review to show the progression of research in an area. When landmark studies are replicated, the literature review should follow the line of research (Galvan, 1999).

Lack of Publications on Topic

The author sometimes may not locate any relevant literature about a topic. Galvan (1999) cautions against writing, "No studies were found." He recommends instead that authors justify these gaps in the literature by explaining how they arrived at this conclusion, such as by indicating what databases were searched, the years searched, other limitations placed on the search, and the search terms.

Grouping Publications

In the synthesis of the literature, studies were grouped, and similarities and differences across them were noted. This is how the literature should be presented rather than listing and discussing each publication separately. The following example demonstrates this principle:

> Many factors affect demand for registered nurses (RNs), including demographics, economic conditions, health care standards, and new technology (Buerhaus, 1998). Between 1983 and 1989, RN employment in U.S. hospitals increased by 13% (Anderson & Wootton, 1991). In the 1990s, journalists reported the use of RNs in hospitals decreased, and demand for nursing personnel declined (Kunen, 1996; Rosenthal, 1996; Shuit, 1996). However, researchers found that the number of hours worked by RNs per hospital and per patient day increased in the early 1990s in California (Anderson & John, 1996; Spetz, 1998).
>
> —Coffman & Spetz, 1999, p. 390

There are seven different articles cited in this literature review, but rather than discussing each one separately, the authors provide two perspectives of the demand for and use of RNs in hospitals: journalists who reported a decrease compared with researchers who found an increase.

When findings are inconsistent, though, the author should report studies separately so as to be clear to readers. For instance, in the following original example, it is not clear which studies had a low return rate of 25% and which had the higher rate of return (65%) after sending reminder postcards.

Original:

Previous studies have shown a return rate of surveys ranging from 25% to 65% after clinic staff sent postcards reminding patients to send back their surveys (Adams, 1998; Gabow, 1999; Smith, 2000).

Revised:

Previous studies have shown a return rate of surveys ranging from 25% (Adams, 1998; Smith, 2000) to 65% after clinic staff sent postcards reminding patients to send back their surveys (Gabow, 1999).

Accuracy of References

Studies have documented errors in journal article reference lists in nursing literature (Foreman & Kirchhoff, 1987; Schulmeister, 1998; Taylor, 1998); in medical journals (Benning & Speer, 1993; Evans, Nadjari, & Burchell, 1990; Orlin, Pehling, Pogrel, 1996); and in veterinary journals (Hinchcliff, Bruce, Powers, & Kipp, 1993). Of 180 references in three nursing journals reviewed by Schulmeister (1998), 58 (32%) had citation errors. Of these, 43 were major errors, making retrieval of the publication difficult.

Reference lists of publications provide a means of evaluating the quality of the articles because they reflect the thoroughness of the author's literature review (Schulmeister, 1998). They also allow others to retrieve publications. Errors in authors' names, journal names, pages numbers, and year of publication may inhibit retrieval of articles and may prevent giving credit to authors for their work. Therefore, accuracy is important with the citations in the literature review, in which many publications often are cited, and on the reference list. Each reference should be checked carefully for errors.

SUMMARY

A literature review is a critique and summary of current knowledge about a topic for research and for use in clinical practice, teaching, administration, and other areas of nursing. Literature reviews are conducted when writing a paper for a course, a thesis, a dissertation, grants, projects in which the nurse may be involved, and manuscripts.

There are three main purposes of reviewing the literature. The first purpose is to describe what is known already about a topic. The literature review provides the background needed for developing a research study, answering questions about clinical practice, developing new projects, and making other decisions. It reveals existing knowledge about a topic and related areas. The second purpose is to identify gaps in knowledge and where questions remain. The third purpose is to determine how the proposed study, project, or paper will contribute new knowledge to nursing.

The author first identifies the topic of the paper and then searches the literature. There are varied bibliographic databases for conducting literature searches in nursing. The two databases that are most useful are MEDLINE and CINAHL.

Each article in a bibliographic database is indexed similarly. It has a single record with specific information about that article. The record has fields, which include information such as the author's name, title of the article, journal in which published, publication date and information, and terms or phrases that describe the content of the article. MeSH is used for MEDLINE indexing and other databases produced by the NLM. CINAHL has its own controlled vocabulary thesaurus based on MeSH but with additional terms for nursing and allied health literature.

After choosing the topic and narrowing it down, the next step is to select the most appropriate database for the search. The author does a preliminary search to evaluate the effectiveness of the search terms. Searches can be modified by choosing other terms to search; by manipulating the fields such as limiting publication dates; and by using the Boolean connectors *and*, *or*, and *not*. These connectors indicate how the computer should combine the search terms and treat them in relation to one another.

The literature should be reviewed starting with the most recent references and working backward. Reference lists of articles, chapters and books also can be examined to identify citations that might have been missed.

The author should keep a record of (1) each database searched, (2) terms used for the search, (3) years searched, (4) limitations placed on the search, and (5) resulting citations. Considering the numerous references retrieved in a search, authors need efficient ways of managing these references and retrieving them for research, writing, and other projects.

Authors need to critically examine each publication before using it as a basis for their own research and writing. Not every document retrieved from a literature review may be used for preparing a manuscript. Some papers are not used because of poor quality; other times, the content is not relevant to the paper. When multiple studies exist in an area, authors can synthesize the literature, noting similarities and consistent findings across studies. This is essential for evidence-based practice.

In writing the literature review, authors should point out how their paper closes a gap in the literature and extends earlier work. They should emphasize how their research replicates an important study and contributes new knowledge to nursing.

REFERENCES

Allen, M. (1998). Selecting keywords: Helping others find your article. *Nurse Author and Editor, 8(*1), 4, 7–9.

Allen, M. (1999). Nursing knowledge access via bibliographic databases. In L.Q. Thede, Computers in nursing: Bridges to the future (pp. 149–170). Philadelphia: Lippincott Williams & Wilkins.

Benning, S.P., & Speer, S.C. (1993). Incorrect citations: A comparison of library literature with medical literature. *Bulletin of the Medical Library Association, 81*, 56–58.

Beyea, S., & Nicoll, L.H. (1998). Writing an integrative review. *AORN Journal*, 67, 877–880.

Burnham, J., & Shearer, B. (1993). Comparison of CINAHL, EMBASE, and MEDLINE databases for the nurse researcher. *Medical Reference Services Quarterly, 12*(3); 45–57.

Burns, N., & Grove, S.K. (1999). *Understanding nursing research* (2nd ed.). Philadelphia: WB Saunders.

CINAHL Information Systems. (2000). The CINAHL® database. [On-line]. Available: *http://www.cinahl.com/prodsvcs/prodsvcs.html*. Accessed June 8, 2000.

Coffman, J., & Spetz, J. (1999). Maintaining an adequate supply of RNs in California. *Image: Journal of Nursing Scholarship, 31*, 389–393.

Evans, J.T., Nadjari, H.I., & Burchell, S.A. (1990). Quotational and reference accuracy in surgical journals. *Journal of the American Medical Association, 263*, 1353–1354.

Foreman, M.D., & Kirchhoff, K.T. (1987). Accuracy of references in nursing journals. *Research in Nursing and Health, 10,* 177–183.

Fosbinder, D., & Loveridge, C. (1996). How to critique a research study. *Advanced Practice Nursing Quarterly, 2*(3), 68–71.

Galvan, J.L. (1999). Writing literature reviews. Los Angeles: Pyrczak Publishing.

Heinrich, K.T. (2000). How long should the literature search be? *Nurse Author & Editor, 10*(1), 1–3.

Hinchcliff, K.W., Bruce, N.J., Powers, J.D., & Kipp, M.L. (1993). Accuracy of references and quotations in veterinary journals. *Journal of the American Veterinary Medical Association, 202*(3), 397–400.

ISI Research Soft. (2000). Software to simplify your research. [On-line]. Available: *http://www.risinc.com*. Accessed June 16, 2000.

Martin, P.A. (1997). Writing a useful literature review for a quantitative research project. *Applied Nursing Research, 10,* 159–162.

National Library of Medicine. (2000a). Fact Sheet. MEDLINE®. [On-line]. Available: *http://www.nlm.nih.gov/pubs/factsheets/medline.html*. Accessed June 13, 2000.

National Library of Medicine. (2000b). Fact sheet: Medical Subject Headings (MeSH). [On-line]. Available: *http://www.nlm.nih.gov/pubs/factsheets/mesh.html*. Accessed June 7, 2000.

Orlin, W., Pehling, J., & Pogrel, M.A. (1996). Do authors check their references? *Journal of Oral and Maxillofacial Surgery, 54,* 200–202.

Rosswurm, M.A., & Larrabee, J.H. (1999). A model for change to evidence-based practice. *Image: Journal of Nursing Scholarship, 31,* 317–322.

Sandelowski, M. (1998). Writing a good read: Strategies for re-presenting qualitative data. *Research in Nursing & Health, 21,* 375–382.

Schulmeister, L. (1998). Quotation and reference accuracy of three nursing journals. *Image: Journal of Nursing Scholarship, 30,* 143–146.

Schwarz, J.K. (1999). Assisted dying and nursing practice. *Image: Journal of Nursing Scholarship, 31,* 367–373.

Taylor, M.K. (1998). The practical effects of errors in reference lists in nursing research journals. *Nursing Research, 47,* 300–303.

Zaruba, K.E., Toma, J.D., & Stark, J.S. (1996). Criteria used for qualitative research in the refereeing process. *The Review of Higher Education, 19,* 435–460.

WRITING RESEARCH ARTICLES

6

Research papers present the findings of quantitative and qualitative research. They may be written for journals that publish mainly research articles, or they may be prepared for clinical journals that report research in that practice specialty. This chapter guides the author in writing research papers. The chapter begins with a discussion of how to report research using the conventional format of introduction, literature review, which may be incorporated into the introduction, methods, results, and discussion. When developing research papers for clinical journals, this format may not be explicit, but it is a framework for the author to use in deciding how to organize the content.

The chapter does not explain the research process or different types of research that might be reported in the literature. Instead, it offers general principles for writing research papers. The author needs to adapt these principles for the type of journal to which the manuscript is submitted.

WHY WRITE ABOUT RESEARCH?

Research projects are not complete until the findings are communicated to others. Often, nurses conduct important research studies but fail to disseminate the results of their work. Some nurses are not prepared for their role as an author and are unsure how to proceed. Others believe that their work does not warrant publication, but "good" research is important to communicate to others, even when the findings were not anticipated. Findings that do not support the hypothesis may be as important as ones that do, since other researchers and clinicians need this information as they plan studies and make decisions about clinical practice.

There are many reasons for disseminating the results of research in the literature. First, nursing research is of little value if the findings are not made available for use by clinicians and others who need the research results for their work. Nurses who conduct research are responsible for reporting the results in journals that are read by nurses who can use the information in their practice, teaching, management, and other roles. Research findings must be disseminated for them to have an effect on patient care and service delivery (Hicks, 1995).

Second, by publishing the findings of research, nurses advance the body of knowledge of nursing and contribute to the scientific basis of nursing practice. Research is essential for professional practice because it generates the knowledge that defines that practice.

Third, communicating the findings of research promotes the critique and replication of studies (Lyder, 1999). Researchers can build studies on one another, extending what is known about the topic and enabling nurses to apply findings to other groups and settings. By reading research reports, nurses also ask new questions that lead to further studies.

Fourth, disseminating the findings of research is essential for research utilization in nursing. Research utilization is the process by which knowledge from research is incorporated into clinical practice (Nicoll & Beyea, 1999). Although research utilization models vary, they all involve the critique of research findings and subsequent use of those findings in practice.

Nurses also need research data to establish evidence for their decisions and interventions. Evidence-based practice involves the use of the best evidence available for making decisions about patient care (McPheeters & Lohr, 1999). This evidence includes clinically relevant research combined with individual clinical expertise. In the model of evidence-based practice by Rosswurm and Larrabee (1999), changes in practice are derived from a review and critique of related research and synthesis of the research findings. Improving the quality of care requires a commitment to provide nursing care that is based on sound research.

Writing about research is similar to making a reasoned argument: the author's goal is to convince readers that the study is important, the methods were appropriate for examining the problem, the findings are valid, and the implications for practice are consistent with the data. The research report or paper summarizes the study and its purpose, methods, and findings. This report is the document that presents key aspects of the study for readers. Research reports vary in length, ranging from manuscripts, which are about 15 to 20 pages, to master's theses and doctoral dissertations, which are significantly longer, ranging from approximately 50 to 200 pages, depending on the study.

Writing Research Papers for Research Journals

The format for the research report follows the same format as the research process. It begins with an introduction and the purpose of the study, proceeds through a description of its methods and results, and concludes with a discussion of the findings. There are differences though in the extent of detail of the paper across journals. When writing a report for a research journal, the author explains each component of the research study with sufficient detail for others to understand the problem, methods, and findings so that the study can be replicated if desired.

For example, Nesbitt and Heidrich (2000) tested a conceptual model of proposed relationships among physical health limitations, the sense of coherence, illness appraisal, and quality of life of older women. The article was organized using the traditional format of a research report: introduction, method, results, and discussion. In the introduction, the researchers presented an extensive critique of related research on each of the concepts in the model; in the methods section, a description was given of the participants, procedure, and measures; and the results section presented the descriptive findings and model testing, based on complex statistical analyses. The article described in detail each component of the research study and was organized in this same way.

Writing Research Papers for Clinical Journals

The author may decide to prepare the research report for a clinical journal that publishes research in that clinical specialty. In research reports in clinical journals, the literature review usually is less extensive than for a research journal, and there is less discussion on the research methods themselves. Readers of clinical journals may not be interested in elaborate discussions of the statistical analyses used in the study, nor would they have the background to understand this discussion. Instead, their focus is on how the research findings can guide their nursing practice. These manuscripts should emphasize the clinical implications of the study. As discussed in earlier chapters, the author needs to gear the paper to the journal and audience.

Antle (2000) developed a research report for *Dimensions of Critical Care Nursing* on nurses repositioning pulmonary artery (PA) catheters. After a brief introduction, the author reviewed the literature on nurses removing and repositioning PA catheters, whether institutions had written protocols for this, complications of PA catheter use, and how to recognize the migration of PA catheters. The literature review included a few research studies and descriptive articles about PA catheters and their maintenance. In the next section of the manuscript, Antle described the development of guidelines for PA catheter repositioning at her medical center and presented them in a table. The remaining section of the research report included the results of her study, conducted over a 2-month period with 125 patients; the discussion; future considerations for research and clinical practice; and recommendations for changes in the guidelines, documentation by nurses, and care of patients with PA catheters. While the research format is apparent in the article, the emphasis is placed on clinical practice implications, and content is included to improve nurses' competency in carrying out this procedure.

For some research projects, the author might write about the research itself for one journal and the implications for practice for a clinical journal. The clinical manuscript then would build on the research report by presenting how the findings can be used by nurses. In this situation, the author references the research report in the clinical manuscript so that readers can obtain details about the study (MacLean, 1999).

Writing About Other Types of Research Projects

The research to be reported in the literature does not have to involve complex studies with large samples. Many studies have been done by nurses on a smaller scale that are important for others to know about. The knowledge gained from evaluations done by nurses of interventions and new initiatives for patients, for instance, may be important for advancing nursing practice and answering questions about clinical practice. Reports of clinical studies conducted in one setting may guide practice by nurses in another setting and may contribute to a better understanding about care of patients. Researchers then can build on these individual studies to develop nursing knowledge.

A good example of a research report of a pilot study was written by Paul (2000). In this article, Paul presented the effects of a multidisciplinary, outpatient heart failure clinic on the clinical and economic management of patients with congestive heart failure. Although only 15 patients were studied, the research builds on earlier projects, described in the literature review, and clearly extends this line of research.

There are other situations in which the author initiated a research study, but because of problems in implementation, was not able to carry it out as planned. In developing a manuscript about the study, the author might view it as a pilot to inform others about its purpose and provide a basis for subsequent research. The author also might develop a manuscript on the difficulties encountered in conducting this type of study and possible solutions.

Perhaps the study provided data to identify the need for a change in nursing practice, to establish a quality improvement project, or to modify the delivery of care. The manuscript in these instances may avoid the conventional format of the research report and instead be developed around the problem that led to the project, a description of the project and data collected, the findings, and the implications for practice. If changes were subsequently made in practice, then the manuscript also may describe these changes and the evaluation planned to monitor them over time. In manuscripts such as these, the research process may guide the author in deciding on content to include and how to organize it, but the manuscript may not be developed using the conventional format of a research report.

For example, Brown (2000) presented the results of a study to increase institutional commitment to improving pain management in two rural hospitals. The study had four goals: (1) to conduct an assessment of the knowledge and attitudes of nurses and other health professionals about pain management, (2) to design a curriculum to educate providers on pain management, (3) to implement a comprehensive pain management program, and (4) to evaluate its effectiveness. The article is organized as follows:

- Initiation of the project
  Assessment phase
  Results of the assessment phase
- Design of pain management program
  Implementation of action plan
  Evaluation of project
- Outcome analysis and recommendations.

Instead of organizing the manuscript using the conventional format of introduction, methods, results, and discussion, the author describes the need for the study and how it was assessed, the educational intervention and its implementation, and the survey results for evaluating its effectiveness. This study would not have been described adequately if the author used a conventional research format. The research process, though, still is apparent in the article.

TITLE

Every research paper needs a title. The title should be carefully worded to capture the objective of the study. The intent of the title is to inform readers what information will be presented in the paper. Key words that represent this content should be used in the title; this draws the attention of readers who are scanning journals or conducting literature searches for relevant articles. For the same reason, the most important words should be listed first.

One title may be written, or it may be developed with a subtitle that provides more specific information about the paper. When subtitles are used, the most important terms should be placed in the title. For example:

Single title

Effectiveness of Different Medication Management Approaches on Elders' Medication Adherence (Winland-Brown & Valiante, 2000)

Title with subtitle

    Elders' Medication Adherence: Effectiveness of Different Medication Management Approaches

Either way, the title communicates the purpose of the study reported in the paper.

Titles should be informative but also concise. Byrne (1998) recommended limiting the title to 10 to 12 words only and avoiding unnecessary phrases such as "a study of" and "an investigation into." By reading the title, the information conveyed in the article should be apparent.

 ## ABSTRACT

Abstracts are more important than titles in directing readers to articles. The abstract provides a summary of the research. It describes the study purpose and background, methods used for the research, and findings. The abstract may be the author's only chance to convince readers that the research is important enough to read the article (MacLean, 1999).

In some journals, structured abstracts are required, and the journals specify the information to be included with labels for the headings. Structured abstracts may include the following headings:

- Purpose
- Design
- Setting
- Subjects
- Measures
- Results
- Conclusions.

Abstracts of an original research report typically are between 120 (American Psychological Association [APA], 1994) to no more than 250 words (American Medical Association [AMA], 1998), although journals often specify the length and format for their abstracts. How to prepare the abstract for a particular journal is indicated in the author guidelines. If the guidelines do not specify a maximum length, the author should keep to a 250-word limit as few journals would allow longer abstracts.

A second reason for limiting the length of the abstract relates to indexing the article. If the abstract is too long, the complete abstract may not be included in the bibliographic database. For example, in the MEDLINE database, there is a 250-word limit for abstracts of articles less than 10 pages and a 400-word limit for abstracts of articles 10 pages or longer (National Library of Medicine, 2000). If the entire abstract is not included, it indicates that the abstract was truncated, but some important content might be omitted.

Display 6.1 provides examples of abstracts for research reports. The first two examples are structured abstracts; although the third example is unstructured, it provides the same information about the study as the other two. More discussion about writing titles and abstracts for other types of articles is provided in later chapters.

DISPLAY 6.1	**Sample Abstracts**

STRUCTURED ABSTRACT: QUANTITATIVE STUDY

Important Attributes of Quality Health Care: Consumer Perspectives

Abstract

Purpose: Despite extensive research on defining and measuring health care quality, less attention has been given to consumers' perspectives of quality health care. The purposes of this study were to (1) identify the importance to consumers of attributes of health care quality and nursing care quality, and (2) examine their relationship to health status and selected demographic variables.

Design: Exploratory: Consumers (N = 239) were recruited from waiting rooms of clinics and in neighborhoods of a large metropolitan area in the Midwest, which included both urban and suburban populations.

Methods: Participants completed the Quality Health Care Questionnaire (QHCQ) and the SF-36 Health Survey. On the QHCQ, they rated the importance of 27 attributes of health care and nursing care quality. The SF-36 is a 36-item instrument measuring health status in eight general areas.

Findings: The most important indicators of quality nursing care to consumers were as follows: being cared for by nurses who are up-to-date and well informed; being able to communicate with the nurse; spending enough time with the nurse and not feeling rushed during the visit; having a nurse teach about the illness, medications, treatments, and staying healthy; and being able to call a nurse with questions. The lowest importance rating was having an opportunity to be cared for by nurse practitioners. Ratings differed by race, age, years of education, income, and health status.

Conclusions: The study emphasizes the importance that consumers place on teaching by the nurse, particularly among people with less education, lower income levels, and chronic illnesses.[1]

[1]From Oermann, M.H., & Templin, T. (2000). Important attributes of quality health care: Consumer perspectives. *Journal of Nursing Scholarship, 32,* 167. Reprinted by permission of Sigma Theta Tau.

(continued)

| DISPLAY 6.1 | **Sample Abstracts** *(Continued)* |

STRUCTURED ABSTRACT: QUALITATIVE STUDY

Domains of Nursing Intervention After Sudden Cardiac Arrest and Automatic Internal Cardioverter Defibrillator Implantation

Abstract

Purpose: The purpose of the study was to explore individual and family experiences after sudden cardiac arrest and automatic internal cardioverter defibrillator implantation during the first year of recovery. This report specifically addresses the domains of concern expressed and helpful strategies used by participants that are relevant to the development of future intervention programs.

Design: A grounded theory approach was used to gain an understanding of areas of concern of survivors of sudden cardiac arrest and their families that could be used when designing future nursing interventions. Semistructured interviews were conducted with both sudden cardiac arrest survivors and one family member each at five points during the first year of recovery (hospitalization; 1, 3, 6, and 12 months after hospitalization). Participants were asked to identify the specific areas that most concerned them, for which they would like assistance with during the first year. A total of 150 interviews were conducted with 176 hours of data generated.

Setting: The study focused on 10 northwest urban community medical centers and participants' homes within a 50-mile driving distance from the medical centers.

Sample: The sample included 15 survivors of first-time sudden cardiac arrest (13 men, 2 women) and one family member each between the ages of 31 and 72 years.

Results: Domains of concern identified by participants that can be used to design future nursing intervention programs include preventive care, dealing with automatic internal cardioverter defibrillator shocks, emotional challenges, physical changes, activities of daily living, partner relationships, and dealing with health care providers. Suggestions of helpful strategies used by participants during the first year are outlined.

Implications: Domains of concern and helpful strategies identified by participants provide a framework for the development and testing of nursing intervention programs to enhance recovery after sudden cardiac arrest for survivors and their families.[2]

ABSTRACT (PARAGRAPH FORM): QUALITATIVE STUDY

The Patient's Diagnosis: Explanatory Models of Mental Illness

Abstract

The study develops a grounded theory about individuals' perception of their situation of being a psychiatric patient. Thirty-five inpatients (19 men, 16 women), ages 18 to 68, in two psychiatric units of an urban, public facility were interviewed on a biweekly basis from

[2]From Dougherty, C.M., Benoliel, J.Q., & Bellin, C. (2000). Domains of nursing intervention after sudden cardiac arrest and automatic internal cardioverter defibrillator implantation. *Heart & Lung, 29,* 79. Reprinted by permission of Mosby.

(continued)

DISPLAY 6.1   **Sample Abstracts** *(Continued)*

admission to discharge. Data were analyzed using the constant comparative method, and the data indicated that participants used the basic social process of managing self-worth to deal with the stigmatizing social predicament of being a mental patient. Events occurring before admission that shaped their responses were substance abuse, medication noncompliance, and the lack of social capital, which led to norm violations and subsequent hospitalization. Six attribution categories emerged: problem, disease, crisis, punishment, ordination, and violation. Findings support the need for professionals to improve their practice by acknowledging the effects of patients' subjective assessment on their response to hospitalization and by placing more emphasis on assisting patients to deal with the stigmatizing effects of a psychiatric diagnosis.[3]

[3]From Sayre, J. (2000). The patient's diagnosis: Explanatory models of mental illness. *Qualitative Health Research, 10*(1), 71. Reprinted by permission of Sage Publications, © 2000.

 ## IMRAD

The conventional format for writing research papers is the IMRAD format—introduction, methods, results and discussion—or an adaptation of this, depending on the journal and type of research (AMA, 1998; APA, 1994; International Committee of Medical Journal Editors [ICMJE], 1997) (Fig. 6-1). IMRAD provides a way of organizing the paper and specifies in advance the headings for it.

Some authors choose to include a separate section in the paper for the literature review rather than incorporating it in the introduction, and subheadings might be included to highlight more specific components of the research. Even when more specificity is added, this format is helpful because it follows the process used for the research and provides a clear structure for the manuscript. The IMRAD format also is useful in writing research reports for clinical journals, even if the structure is not explicit in the paper.

Questions Answered by IMRAD

The IMRAD format follows the research process and answers four important questions of interest to readers:

- Why was the study done?
- What was done?
- What did the researcher find?
- What does it mean?

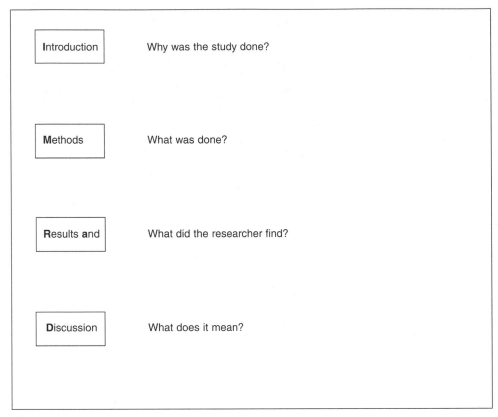

Figure 6-1. IMRAD format.

Why Was the Study Done?

The first question to be answered in the manuscript is why the study was done. A manuscript written for a research or clinical journal should begin with an explanation of the problem and its importance to nursing, leading to the questions that need answers or hypotheses to be tested. Presenting *why* the study was undertaken and its importance is an effective strategy for gaining reader interest in the topic and convincing them to read the article. Answering why the study was done provides the basis for the introduction, which includes information about the background of the study, significance of the research, and questions examined in the study.

What Was Done?

Once the reader understands the problem, its importance, and the purpose of the study, the next question is what did the researcher do? How were the study questions answered or the hypotheses tested? What procedures did the researcher use? This content reflects the methods section of the paper.

What Did the Researcher Find?

Once readers know the problem and how it was studied, the next question is what was learned? What were the findings of the study? In answering these questions, the author presents the data, statistical analyses, observations, and interview results in the results section of the paper. This part of the paper provides the answers to the research questions with supporting evidence.

What Does it Mean?

In this last section of the research paper, the discussion, the researcher answers an important question for readers, "What do these findings mean for clinical practice, teaching, or management, and what do they mean for future research?" This is the section of the paper in which authors discuss their findings and how they compare with other similar studies.

IMRAD Format for Research Papers

Introduction

The first section of the manuscript is the introduction, which is the author's opportunity to explain the nature and background of the study, its purpose, and its importance. The goals of the introductory section are to explain the study to the reader and why it was done.

The author should begin the introduction with a discussion of the specific problem addressed by the research and its significance. This discussion provides a framework for reading the related literature; determining how the study builds on previous research on the topic; and understanding the relationship of the purposes, questions, or hypotheses to the problem. Introducing the problem statement early in the manuscript also clarifies why certain concepts and theories were used to guide the research.

In the beginning sentences, readers should learn what problem was examined in the study and why the research is important to them. When writing for a clinical journal, a good introduction links the significance of the study to the nurse's own clinical practice. This writing not only sets the stage for the remainder of the manuscript, but captures the reader's interest.

When the research project was planned originally, the author reviewed the literature and identified gaps in the research. In the introduction, the author can refer to these gaps in knowledge and how the current study meets these needs. Display 6.2 is an example of an effective introduction because it presents the problem early in the discussion and suggests gaps in the research addressed by the study.

   Sample Introduction

Fever is a common symptom in hospitalized HIV/AIDS patients (Holtzclaw, 1998; Jones, Holloman, & Coffin, 1998). Nurses caring for patients with AIDS use antipyretic medications plus physical cooling methods for fever management (Jones, 1998). However, no studies have evaluated the efficacy of these interventions with patients who have HIV/AIDS. Additionally, no research reports have evaluated the use of a "cooling scarf," a new physical cooling method used by the lay public while exercising, as a method that could be applied in the clinical setting. Therefore, a pilot study was designed to compare three interventions for nursing management of low-grade to moderate fever (100.5° to 104°F) in hospitalized patients with HIV/AIDS. The study determines which intervention was the most effective in decreasing body temperature while increasing patient comfort.

From Jones, S.G. (1999). Pilot testing three interventions for symptom management in HIV/AIDS fever. *Image: Journal of Nursing Scholarship, 31,* 346. Reprinted by permission of Sigma Theta Tau.

Some authors include too much discussion in the background of the study before they identify the specific problem under investigation. Instead, the statement of the problem should be clear to readers in the beginning of the introduction.

Literature Review

The literature review describes what is already known about the topic and what needs to be studied, thereby justifying the current project. The literature review is critical to validate the need for the research (Lyder, 1999). In the literature review, the author synthesizes related research, summarizes major findings from the studies, indicates when they are consistent, and suggests reasons for conflicting results. Gaps in knowledge and limitations of prior studies are emphasized to provide support for the current study. The author also may address methodological issues in the research, particularly when the current study sought to resolve these. How to review the literature and write the literature review was presented in Chapter 5.

Typically, for research papers, only research studies are included in the literature review section. Display 6.3 depicts a portion of a literature review that demonstrates how to organize studies for a research manuscript. Notice that the studies are organized around topics rather than the findings of individual researchers. Descriptive articles, anecdotal reports, and other nonresearch papers may be used in the beginning of the manuscript to introduce the problem, but, generally, only research is incorporated in the literature review.

The intent of the literature review is to present relevant studies that provide the background for the current research and why the study was indicated. It is not an exhaustive review of the research, nor is the author attempting to

| DISPLAY 6.3 | Sample Literature Review |

PURPOSE

This study described and examined relationships among pain, psychological distress, perceived health status, and coping in patients with breast cancer after treatment with mastectomy and chemotherapy before autotransplantation. Assessment of pain, psychological distress, perceived health status, and coping helps health care providers to understand and provide appropriate care for patients during this phase of treatment. This study examined to what degree pain, psychological distress, and coping were predictors of health status.

LITERATURE REVIEW

Research literature exists regarding the pain, psychological distress, and coping experienced by patients undergoing autotransplantation during and after hospitalization (Gaston-Johansson, Franco, & Zimmerman, 1992; Hill et al., 1990; Jenkins & Roberts, 1991). However, there is a paucity of research exploring these variables before autotransplantation. Assessment and treatment of patients' emotional state is extremely important before transplantation procedures and associated intensive chemotherapy because efforts can be directed at reducing psychological distress and helping patients to better cope with the upcoming situation (Gaston-Johansson & Foxall, 1996).

Conceptual Framework

The Gate Control Theory of Pain of Melzack and Wall (1982) and the Stress, Coping, and Adaptation paradigm of Lazarus and Folkman (1984) provided the theoretical framework for this study. Pain is defined as a multidimensional sensory and affective experience associated with discomfort (International Association for the Study of Pain, 1979). According to the Gate Control Theory of Pain, the central system located in the brain can be stimulated by cognitive processes (eg, past experiences, anxiety, anticipation, attention), which open the gating mechanism and permit the transmission of nociceptive impulses to the brain (Melzack & Wall, 1982).

Pain

Several studies have shown that pain was a significant problem for patients with stage I or II breast cancer (Arathuzik, 1991; Miaskowski & Dibble, 1995a, 1995b). Pain may be acute (as experienced before diagnosis and after lumpectomy or mastectomy and axillary node dissection) or chronic and long term (Gorrell, d'Angelo, & Bagley, 1988). Patients with breast cancer have characterized this treatment-related pain as irritating (Gorrell, et al., 1988), shooting, throbbing, burning, stabbing, pulling, and tight (Stevens, Dibble, & Miaskowski, 1995). Only one published study examined the pain that patients with breast cancer experienced and its effects on their lives in the outpatient setting (Miaskowski & Dibble, 1995b). Forty-seven percent of the patients in this study who were receiving treatment in the outpatient setting reported moderate to severe cancer-related pain on a daily basis. Most of these women had treatment-related pain from postsurgical neuropathic pain syndrome (56%) and cancer-related pain from bone metastasis (26%).

(continued)

Patients who experience cancer pain have significantly more depression, anxiety, and decreased quality-of-life scores than pain-free patients (Ferrell, Dow, Leigh, Ly, & Gulasekaram, 1995; Ferrell & Funk, 1995; Miaskowski & Dibble, 1995b). Arathuzik's (1994) pilot study found that educating patients with breast cancer in relaxation techniques and cognitive coping skills was effective in decreasing pain. Used separately, these nonpharmacologic approaches have proven to be effective in relieving pain in patients with breast and lung cancer (Arathuzik, 1994; Ferrell-Torry & Glick, 1993; Wilkie, 1990, 1991). However, these approaches have not been evaluated in combination in a randomized, controlled clinical trial.

Selected part of literature review from Gaston-Johansson, F., Ohly, K.V., Fall-Dickson, J.M., Nanda, J.P., & Kennedy, M.J. (2000). Pain, psychological distress, health status, and coping in patients with breast cancer scheduled for autotransplantation. *Oncology Nursing Forum, 26,* 1338. Adapted by permission of Oncology Nursing Society.

give a historical perspective to the field of study. Readers will gain a sense of the development of the research by reviewing the progression of studies.

Authors must be cognizant of the length of the literature review because of space limitations of the manuscript. Tornquist and Funk (1993) suggest keeping the review of the literature short because readers are more interested in what the researcher did in the study than what the researcher read. Often, in preparing a research grant or writing a thesis or dissertation, extensive literature is reviewed and summarized, some of which may be tangential to the manuscript. Generally, literature reviews for grants, theses, and dissertations need to be rewritten for the manuscript, with references carefully selected. Rarely can these literature reviews be used "as is" for manuscripts.

One additional point is to update the literature review from the time it was originally written because newer studies may have emerged. Some research projects take many years to complete, and the literature review done at the time the research was planned may be out of date when the manuscript is written.

The literature review may be incorporated into the introduction, as suggested by the IMRAD format, or presented as a separate section in the manuscript. This differs across nursing journals. The author should read selected articles in the potential journals to gain a sense of how they handle the literature review.

When writing research reports for clinical journals, the literature review generally is less extensive than for a research journal and often is incorporated into the introduction rather than presented as a separate section. For clinical journals, readers are interested in the purpose and significance of the study and how they may use the findings for their own practice. Generally, they are not interested in comprehensive literature reviews or elaborate discussions on research methods.

Theoretical Framework

The literature review may contain the discussion of the conceptual or theoretical framework that guided the study, or the framework may be included in a separate section. In the example in Display 6.3, the conceptual framework is discussed within the literature review. Presenting the framework is one way of organizing the literature because the framework includes the variables and their relationships that are relevant to the research study (MacLean, 1999).

Display 6.4 provides two examples of a theoretical framework incorporated in the introduction of a research report. The length and complexity of the description of the conceptual or theoretical framework vary across research reports. With some manuscripts, authors discuss the framework in detail, particularly when the research tested a model. In other research reports, often those prepared for clinical journals, the discussion of the framework may be

---

DISPLAY 6.4 Sample Theoretical Frameworks

The theoretical framework of this study was a systems perspective of person–environment interactions and outcomes. The framework included practice environment and nurse personal systems variables thought to contribute to nurses' self-reported willingness to engage in actions to resolve clinical ethical dilemmas. In this framework, nurses' personal characteristics, in combination with characteristics of the practice environment, influence ethical practice outcomes—nurses' willingness to take action to resolve clinical ethical dilemmas. Level of nursing education also was included in the study framework because previous studies suggested a relationship between nurses' levels of education and ethical practice (Ketefian, 1981, 1988).[1]

The framework for the study was a model developed by Kravitz (1996). This model links patient expectations and satisfaction with a medical encounter. In the model, patients' expectations for care are formed before the encounter and include expectations for care in general and for the specific visit. These expectations are influenced by demographic characteristics, prior health care experiences, and concerns related to the patient's specific health problems. Patients evaluate their visit with the provider by comparing the events that occurred with their expectations. An understanding of these expectations is important because meeting them may lead to greater satisfaction with care (Kravitz, 1996).[2]

[1]From Penticuff, J.H., & Walden, M. (2000). Influence of practice environment and nurse characteristics on perinatal nurses' responses to ethical dilemmas. *Nursing Research, 49,* 65. Reprinted by permission of Lippincott Williams & Wilkins.

[2]From Oermann, M.H., & Templin, T. (2000). Important attributes of quality health care: Consumer perspectives. *Journal of Nursing Scholarship, 32,* 167. Reprinted by permission of Sigma Theta Tau.

limited or not included in the manuscript. In the first example in Display 6.5, the author integrates a statement of the theoretical framework with the purpose of the study. Whether to discuss the framework and to what depth depend on the journal, the goal of the paper, and the objective of the research study.

Purpose

The last part of the introduction includes the statement of the purpose of the study: what was done. This should be the closing paragraph of the introduction (APA, 1994). The author may include a statement of the (1) purposes of the study, (2) questions that the research was designed to answer, and (3) hypotheses that were tested. An example of each of these is shown in Display 6.5. A clear statement of the purpose of the research is essential to provide a rationale for the method, which is discussed in the next section of the manuscript.

Huth (1999) suggested that only the main questions be included in the introduction and that subsidiary questions be presented in the results section of the manuscript. For instance, in a study comparing interventions for wound care, the researcher also might have examined the costs of each treatment and number of nursing hours needed to provide care. The main question, though, is the effectiveness of each intervention in promoting wound healing. This main question should be presented in the introduction, keeping the report focused on the effectiveness of those treatments, with other less important questions and answers presented in the results.

The introduction should not contain a statement about the research design or any of the findings. These are presented later in the paper.

Methods

The next section of the manuscript is methods. How did the researcher carry out the study? What was done? In the methods section, information about the study design, subjects, measures, procedures, and data analysis is presented in this order. Often, each subsection is labeled accordingly, making it easy for the reader to follow the methodology of the research.

The methods section needs to be detailed to demonstrate the validity and reliability of the methodology in a quantitative study and trustworthiness in a qualitative study (MacLean, 1999). Detail also is important so that researchers can replicate the study if desired. After writing the methods section, a colleague can be asked to assess whether the description clearly communicates the methods and whether the methods could be replicated with the information provided. When writing research for clinical and nonresearch journals, though, less detail is provided on the methods of the study.

This section is written in past tense because the study has been completed. Often the write-up from the research grant, thesis, or dissertation may be

PURPOSE

A pilot study was designed to compare three interventions for nursing management of low-grade to moderate fever (100.5° to 104°F) in hospitalized patients with HIV/AIDS. The purpose of the study was to determine which intervention was the most effective in decreasing body temperature while increasing patient comfort. The theoretical framework for the study was derived from Kolcaba's (1995) theory of comfort care, in which outcomes of nursing practice are measured by patients' perceptions of their own comfort. The theory can be applied in clinical settings by assessing patients' perceptions of comfort before and after nursing interventions.[1]

RESEARCH QUESTIONS

While research suggests that university nursing faculty experience different levels of role strain and burnout, this research focuses primarily on full-time faculty balancing teaching, research, service, and, in some instances, clinical practice responsibilities. None of the prior studies examined the role of clinical nursing faculty as a group or included clinical teachers from both associate degree and baccalaureate nursing programs. Because of the lack of research on clinical nursing faculty, the questions for this study were (1) What is the degree of role strain among clinical nursing faculty? and (2) Are there differences in role strain based on the educational preparation of the clinical teacher, level of nursing students for whom responsible, and employment status (full and part time)?[2]

HYPOTHESES

The purpose of this study was to evaluate the reliability and validity of two different health outcome measures for assessing the quality of nursing care in a home health setting. The authors hypothesized the following:

H1. Health status measures would be lower for patients with high nursing intensity than for patients with low nursing intensity.

H2. Health status scores would improve significantly from admission to the nursing agency until discharge or within 30 visits, whichever came first.

H3. Health status scores would improve to a greater extent for the acutely ill patients than for either patients receiving palliative care or patients with chronic illness.

H4. Patients who received care consistently from one provider would experience greater improvement in health outcomes than patients who received care from multiple nurse providers.

H5. The proportion of visits made by a registered nurse would be positively associated with improvement in functional health and quality of life outcomes.[3]

[1]From Jones, S.G. (1999). Pilot testing three interventions for symptom management in HIV/AIDS fever. *Image: Journal of Nursing Scholarship, 31,* 346. Reprinted by permission of Sigma Theta Tau.

[2]From Oermann, M.H. (1998). Role strain of clinical nursing faculty. *Journal of Professional Nursing, 14,* 330–331. Reprinted by permission of W.B. Saunders.

[3]From Irvine, D., O'Brien-Pallas, L.L., Murray, M., Cockerill, R., Sidani, S., Laurie-Shaw, B., et al. (2000). The reliability and validity of two health status measures for evaluating outcomes of home care nursing.

used in the manuscript if it is changed to past tense, updated if procedures changed from the original proposal, and shortened, considering the page limits of the manuscript. In research proposals and studies completed as student requirements, the methods section may include a rationale for each component. In the manuscript, though, this rationale is not necessary unless the study addresses methodologic issues or tests new methods for examining the problem.

If the research is an extension of an earlier study, the author can refer the reader to that article for more detailed information about the methodology. An example follows:

> Data were collected by interview and the Quality Health Care Questionnaire (QHCQ). Veterans were asked four-open ended questions on their definitions of nursing care quality and to describe an experience that represented quality care. The QHCQ included 27 attributes of health care and nursing care quality identified from the literature and prior research. This instrument was used in a related study and is described there with examples (Oermann & Templin, 2000).

Design

The first subsection is the study design. This should be consistent with the background of the study and with the purposes, questions, or hypotheses presented in the introduction. For designs that are well known, such as descriptive and experimental, no further information is needed other than indicating the design used for the research. However, new or unusual designs should be described in detail (Huth, 1999). Sample statements of the design are found in Display 6.6.

For intervention studies, it should be clear to the reader how the study groups were determined and how the interventions differed across the groups. An example of this is seen in Display 6.6.

For qualitative manuscripts, the method of the study, such as grounded theory, phenomenology, ethnography, and historical research, would be described. Display 6.6 includes an example from an article on a qualitative study.

Subjects

The next subsection deals with the subjects who were studied. The description of the participants in the research is important for making comparisons across groups, generalizing the findings, and replicating the study (APA, 1994). Results can be interpreted accurately only when there is sufficient information provided about who was studied and their characteristics.

Sample Design Statements

QUANTITATIVE STUDY

A cross-sectional, descriptive, correlational design was used. Participants were recruited by nonprobability methods within a four-county region from two bordering midwestern states. Inclusion criteria specified English-speaking women aged 65 or older, who live at home, report having at least one chronic health problem, and whose mental status allows reliable participation in the interview process.[1]

INTERVENTION STUDY

An experimental design was used with three study groups representing different approaches for managing medication administration at home: (1) a pillbox method, (2) a voice-activated method, and (3) self-administration of medications. Subjects were randomly assigned to one of these groups. In the pillbox method, individual doses were stored, and the pillbox was prefilled on a weekly basis. The voice-activated method audibly reminded and automatically dispensed individual doses of medication to the subject. The self-administration group served as the control group, with subjects dispensing their own medications.[2]

QUALITATIVE STUDY

The meanings of menopause among a vulnerable group of women—low-income Korean immigrants—were explored using a cross-sectional descriptive research design focusing on how these meanings were constructed with their daily life experiences. Qualitative methods used were in-depth interviews guided by feminist approaches. Feminist approaches respect women's own views and experiences and emphasize the constructions of gender and cultural responses to menopause (Fee, 1983; Hall & Stevens, 1991; Rosser, 1994).[3]

[1]From Nesbitt, B.J., & Heidrich, S.M. (2000). Sense of coherence and illness appraisal in older women's quality of life. *Research in Nursing & Health, 23,* 27. Reprinted by permission of John Wiley & Sons, Inc.
[2]From Winland-Brown, J.E., & Valiante, J. (2000). Effectiveness of different medication management approaches on elders' medication adherence. *Outcomes Management for Nursing Practice, 4,* 172–176. Reprinted by permission of Lippincott Williams & Wilkins.
[3]From Im, E-O., & Meleis, A.I. (2000). Meanings of menopause to Korean immigrant women. *Western Journal of Nursing Research, 22,* 84, 86. Reprinted by permission of Sage Publications, Inc. © 2000.

In writing the description of the subjects, the author can refer to the following list for information that may be included in this section, depending on the type of study:

- Source of subjects
- Number of subjects recruited, number who participated, and number in each study group if relevant
- How subjects were recruited

- Criteria for including and excluding participants
- How subjects were assigned within the study
- Randomization method if random assignment was used
- Basis for decisions about sample size
- Procedures when subjects withdrew from study and actions taken, including how many and why
- Payments made to subjects.

In Display 6.7, the sample is described in the beginning of the methods section to give the reader an understanding of patients who participated in the research. Demographic information about the subjects, such as age, gender, racial and ethnic background, and educational level, usually is reported in the beginning of the results section of the manuscript, particularly when these are variables in the study. This is what the researchers did in the study presented in Display 6.7. The results of that study are summarized in Display 6.10; notice that the first section of the results is a description of the sample characteristics.

An explanation should be included about human subject requirements met for the research. This includes a statement about informed consent, review and approval of the research proposal by the institutional review board, and its review and approval by the institutions where the subjects were recruited. Frequently, one statement suffices, such as, "The study was approved by the institutional review boards of the university and participating hospitals before subject selection. Each subject signed an informed consent." For other studies, though, more information may need to be provided.

Interventions

For intervention studies, the groups and treatments can be described as part of the design, such as in the second example in Display 6.6. However, for some studies, more explanation is needed. In this instance, a section can be added to the report that describes the interventions in more detail (Display 6.8). This is important when writing research papers for clinical journals because readers are interested in new interventions designed to enhance patient care (Tornquist & Funk, 1993). They need to be told in the paper what was done and how so that they can compare the intervention to their own practice and setting.

Tornquist and Funk (1993) offer these suggestions when writing about an intervention study. The author should explain the following:

- What was done and the order
- How long it took
- Who did it

METHODS

Design

The study used a descriptive, correlational design. Inclusion criteria included patients with stage II, III, or IV breast cancer who previously had been treated with mastectomy and chemotherapy and were scheduled to receive an autotransplantation, who were aged 18 years or older and had the ability to speak and read English. The setting was an urban National Cancer Institute–designated comprehensive cancer center located in the eastern United States. The institutional review board approved the study before participant accrual. Each participant signed an informed consent.

Instruments

The **Sociodemographic Questionnaire** gathered information regarding age, gender, race/ethnicity, marital status, educational level, religion, living arrangements, average yearly household income, occupation, work status, and breast cancer stage as verified by the medical record.

The **Gaston-Johansson Painometer**® (1996) was designed to assess patients' overall pain intensity and intensity of sensory and affective components of pain, as well as the quality of pain. The Painometer is a hard, white, plastic tool that measures 8 inches long, 2 inches wide, and 1 inch thick. It is lightweight and easy for participants to hold. The front of the Painometer lists 15 sensory and 11 affective pain descriptors, and a 100-mm visual analogue scale (VAS) with a moveable marker (Painometer-VAS) is located on the back. An intensity value (from a low of 1 to a high of 5) is predetermined for each sensory and affective word located on the Painometer-Words. The maximum score for the sensory component of pain is 36, and for the affective component, the maximum is 34. To obtain a total score, add the sensory and affective scores.

High correlations were found between the initial and the repeat pain intensity ratings on the Painometer-VAS ($r = .88$, $p < .001$) and Painometer-Words ($r = .84$, $p < .001$) (test–retest reliability). Correlations among the Painometer-Words, the McGill Pain Questionnaire ($r = .69$, $p < .001$), and the Painometer-VAS ($r = .84$, $p < .001$) support the concurrent validity of the Painometer-Words. Construct validity was supported for the Painometer by showing that pain scores decreased significantly for the Painometer-Words ($t = 5.53$ $p < .001$) and Painometer-VAS ($t = 6.18$, $p < .001$) after treatment with pain medication. The Painometer takes about 2 minutes to complete.

Psychological distress was measured using the **State-Trait Anxiety Inventory** (STAI) (Spielberger, Gorsuch, & Lushene, 1971) and the **Beck Depression Inventory** (BDI, 1970). The STAI, an extensively used measure of anxiety, consists of two separate self-report scales for measuring state and trait anxiety. Each scale consists of 20 statements that participants rate regarding how they feel in general (trait) and at one particular moment in time (state). Respondents rate themselves in relation to each statement on a Likert-type scale, with score anchors ranging from 1 (not at all) to 4 (very much so). The total score is the sum of all responses, with 20 to 39 = low anxiety, 40 to 59 = moderate anxiety, and 60 to 80 = high anxiety. Spielberger et al. report test–retest reliability coefficients of .73 to .86 and .86 to .92 for the trait subscale and coefficients of .16 to .54 and .83 to .92 for the state subscale. Alpha coefficients estimating internal consistency ranged from .83 to .92 for state and .86 to .92 for trait anxiety.

(continued)

The BDI was used to measure depression. Subjects responded to a Likert-type scale by rating each item 0 (no symptom) to 3 (severe or persistent presence of the symptom). The total score (0 to 63) is obtained by summing the 21 responses with the following interpretations: 0 to 9 = normal, 10 to 15 = mild depression, 16 to 23 = moderate depression, and 24 to 63 = severe depression. The alpha coefficient for the BDI was reported to be .84 to .86, with a Spearman-Brown coefficient of .93.

The **Coping Strategy Questionnaire (CSQ),** developed by Keefe et al. (1987), assessed patients' use of coping strategies. For each category of coping strategies, six items are listed on the CSQ, with possible total scores ranging from 0 to 36. Each item is rated on a seven-point scale to indicate how often that strategy is used to cope with pain (0 = never, 3 = sometimes, and 6 = always). CSQ reliability has been demonstrated with alpha coefficients ranging from .71 to .85. Cronbach's alpha ranged from .71 to .88 in patients receiving chemotherapy. Construct validity was demonstrated by factor analysis (Carey & Burish, 1987; Keefe et al., 1990).

The **Medical Outcomes Study Short-Form General Health Survey (MOS-SF)** (Stewart et al., 1988) was used to measure perceived health status. This 20-item survey assessed physical functioning (six items), role functioning (two items), social functioning (one item), mental health (five items), health perception (five items), and pain (one item) (Stewart et al.). Construct validity was demonstrated by showing that poor health was significantly greater ($p < .001$) in a patient sample than a general population sample regarding physical and role functioning, mental health, and health perceptions.

Procedures

All participants were recruited by either the physician co-investigator or the bone marrow transplant (BMT) clinical nurse specialist co-investigator during a regularly scheduled pre-autotransplantation outpatient clinic visit. All participants had been accepted into the autotransplantation program before receiving an invitation to participate in this study.

The subjects completed the questionnaires in a quiet, comfortable room located in the outpatient clinic. The BMT clinical nurse specialist provided the baseline questionnaires, clarified directions for completion, and retrieved the questionnaires from the participants. Subjects took approximately 1 hour to complete the questionnaires.

Data Analysis

Measures of central tendency were used to describe the sample and responses to the instrument. Correlations among pain intensity, psychological distress, coping variables, and perceived health status were examined using Pearson product moment and Spearman rho correlations, as appropriate. Hierarchical multiple linear regression techniques were used to determine the best fit model that explained the maximum variance of total health status within the context of the study.

Selected part of methods from Gaston-Johansson, F., Ohly, K.V., Fall-Dickson, J.M., Nanda, J.P., & Kennedy, M.J. (2000). Pain, psychological distress, health status, and coping in patients with breast cancer scheduled for autotransplantation. *Oncology Nursing Forum, 26,* 1339–1341. Adapted by permission of Oncology Nursing Society.

| DISPLAY 6.8 | **Sample Descriptions of Interventions** |

EDUCATIONAL INTERVENTION

The intervention used to fill the waiting time in the clinic was videotape instruction on the health condition of the patient population seen in the clinic combined with interaction with the nurse. The videotape was preceded by a brief, verbal explanation by the nurse on (1) the purpose of the videotape, (2) why the instruction is important to the patient's health care and maintaining health, (3) specific learning outcomes to be met from viewing the videotape while waiting in the clinic, and (4) key points to remember. After viewing of the videotape, the nurse provided an opportunity for patients to ask questions about the content in the videotape. The same nurse conducted all the educational interventions.

CLINICAL INTERVENTION

The interventions were (1) oral administration of acetaminophen (Tylenol, 650 mg)—antipyretic without a physical cooling method; (2) Tylenol plus the application of a cooling scarf (the CoolDana bandana scarf, Personal Comfort Corp., Orlando, FL) wrapped around the neck for 1 hour—antipyretic with a physical cooling method; and (3) Tylenol plus the application of cool compresses to the forehead, reapplied every 15 minutes for 1 hour—antipyretic with a different physical cooling method. Evaluation was patients' self-reports of their perception of comfort by use of a Visual Analog Scale (VAS); comparison of temperature (using the CoreCheck® tympanic thermometer), pulse, respiration, and blood pressure; and oxygen saturation rate (obtained using a Nellcor® bedside pulse oximeter and fingertip electrode) before and 1 hour after each intervention.[1]

[1]From Jones, S.G. (1999). Pilot testing three interventions for symptom management in HIV/AIDS fever. *Image: Journal of Nursing Scholarship, 31,* 346. Reprinted by permission of Sigma Theta Tau.

- What kind of training was needed before the intervention and how it was implemented
- If the intervention was theoretically based
- Each intervention, if multiple ones were used, and the control group, if included in the study.

Measures

In the next subsection, the author describes the measures used for the study. This includes a discussion of the instruments, observations, and other measures for collecting the data. The author should include a description of the validity and reliability of each measure, and for previously unpublished measures, the author should explain how they were validated. If the research involved the use of equipment, this should be indicated, including its manufacturer.

Display 6.7 presents the methods section from the study by Gaston-Johansson, Ohly, Fall-Dickson, Nanda, and Kennedy (2000) on pain, psychological distress, coping, and health status in patients with breast cancer. It is easy to see how the researchers collected data for this study and how the instruments relate to the purposes of the research. Notice the consistency between the purposes (See Display 6.3), organization of the literature, and order used to present the instruments. This type of organization is essential in a research report so that readers can see the relationships among the components of the study.

Qualitative manuscripts emphasize methods and sources of data collection, such as interviews and field notes, and how these data were recorded, transcribed, and then analyzed.

Procedures

In the procedures subsection, the author presents each step in carrying out the research. This includes how surveys were distributed to subjects and returned to the investigator, how instruments and other measures were administered to subjects, the explanations given to participants, how groups were formed and interventions implemented, and other steps in collecting the data and carrying out the research. The principle for writing the procedures section is to describe what was done in enough detail for others to replicate it. The procedures used in the study by Gaston-Johansson, Ohly, Fall-Dickson, Nanda, and Kennedy (2000) are in Display 6.7.

Data Analysis

The final subsection in methods deals with the statistical procedures used for data analysis. In this section, the author lists the statistical methods, the alpha level considered acceptable, how variables were selected and analyzed, and computer programs used for the analysis. The goal of this section is to explain to readers how the data were analyzed. For some research reports, often of studies that used known statistical methods, the author may choose not to include a separate subsection on data analysis methods because these are indicated with the results.

Display 6.9 provides examples of data analysis sections. In the first example, from a quantitative study, the statistical methods are listed for the reader; because these are common procedures, no further discussion is indicated. The second example is from a qualitative study. Often in qualitative reports, the author provides a detailed explanation of how the data were analyzed, what software program was used for organizing the analysis, coding strategies, how saturation was determined, and how the validity and reliability of the data were addressed. For qualitative studies, authors need to describe the analytic approach (Polit & Hungler, 1997).

| DISPLAY 6.9 | **Sample Statements of Data Analysis** |

QUANTITATIVE STUDY

Data were analyzed using descriptive statistics. Pearson correlation was used to examine the relationships among age, number of chronic health problems, scores on the Quality Health Care Questionnaire (QHCQ), and SF-36 scores. Differences in scores on the QHCQ between subjects cared for by nurse practitioners and physicians were examined using t tests.

QUALITATIVE STUDY

Grounded theory provided the basis for the qualitative data generation and analysis. Interviews were audiotape recorded and transcribed verbatim. Data were entered into the Non-numerical Unstructured Data Indexing Searching and Theorizing (NUD*IST) program for organizing the analysis. Constant comparative analysis was used as an ongoing technique, which included deriving first-level codes at each time period, comparing codes, deriving conceptual categories, and then relating categories to codes and to other categories.

Validity and reliability of the data were addressed systematically by use of the criteria outlined by Sandelowski (1986) and Lincoln and Guba (1985): (1) credibility, (2) transferability, (3) dependability, and (4) confirmability. Coding of the data was completed by one independent investigator; then, reliability checks were conducted with a second investigator. Techniques of debriefing between peers, member checks, triangulation, prolonged engagement with the data, reflective journals, summaries, persistent observation, and the use of extensive memos were used for ensuring validity and reliability.[1]

[1]From Dougherty, C.M., Benoliel, J.Q., & Bellin, C. (2000). Domains of nursing intervention after sudden cardiac arrest and automatic internal cardioverter defibrillator implantation. *Heart & Lung, 29,* 81. Reprinted by permission of Mosby.

Results

In the results section, the author presents the findings of the study. What was learned from this research? What new evidence was gathered? The findings should address the original purposes of the study and should answer each of the research questions. This is the section in which the author presents the data and its analysis but without discussion of the findings. The discussion is held for the subsequent section. The reader needs an understanding of the results before considering their relationship to previous research and their implications. An example of how to present the results is found in Display 6.10.

The author is obligated to present all of the findings, even when they run counter to what was anticipated and do not support the hypotheses. In these cases, the author examines, in the discussion section, possible reasons for the findings.

Sample Results

RESULTS

Sample Characteristics

The convenience sample of 83 female patients with breast cancer who were scheduled for autotransplantation was composed primarily of white women who were well educated, married, and employed in professional occupations with an average yearly household income of more than $50,000. Data regarding the date of mastectomy and adjuvant chemotherapy were not obtained. Table 1 presents the demographic characteristics of the sample.

Pain

Fifty-four percent of the participants experienced no pain. All mean pain intensity scores were low (Table 2). Although the mean pain scores were low for sensory, affective, overall intensity, and the Painometer-VAS, the range of reported scores was wide. This indicated that some subjects did experience moderate pain intensity.

Study participants experienced pain primarily in the vagina (19%), chest (14%), shoulder (13%), and arm (10%) (Table 3). The words most frequently chosen to describe the sensory quality of pain were aching (25%), sore (24%), and dull (13%), and the words most frequently chosen to describe the affective quality of pain were annoying (26%), tiring (17%), nagging (10%), and troublesome (10%) (Table 4).

Psychological Distress

The participants reported a range of mild (49%) to severe/high (26%) state anxiety ($M = 41.43$, $SD = 12.67$). Forty percent of the sample experienced no depression, with a range of mild (36%) to severe/high (7%) depression reported ($M = 11.66$, $SD = 7.73$).

Cognitive Coping Strategies

The subjects used a variety of coping strategies to deal with pain (Table 5). Positive coping strategies (eg, coping statements, praying, hoping, and diverting attention) were used frequently. Overall, the results demonstrated that participants experienced a moderate ability to control and decrease pain.

Health Status

Subjects reported a mean total perceived health status rating of 50.30 ($SD = 10.67$) of a possible total rating of 0 to 91. The highest mean rating was reported for mental health ($M = 22.10$, $SD = 4.5$). The lowest mean was reported for role functioning ($M = 0.79$, $SD = 0.87$).

Correlations Among Selected Variables and Predictors of Health Status

Table 6 presents correlations among pain, anxiety, depression, coping, and health status. Significant correlations were observed between state anxiety and depression ($r = .61$, $p < .001$) and physical functioning and role functioning ($r = .65$, $p < .001$). Pain, anxiety, depression, and ability to control pain all were significantly correlated to total health status.

Selected part of results from Gaston-Johansson, F., Ohly, K.V., Fall-Dickson, J.M., Nanda, J.P., & Kennedy, M.J. (2000). Pain, psychological distress, health status, and coping in patients with breast cancer scheduled for autotransplantation. *Oncology Nursing Forum, 26,* 1341, 1343. Adapted by permission of Oncology Nursing Society.

Describe Subjects

With some manuscripts, the participants in the study may be described adequately in the method, allowing the author to begin the results with the findings related to the research questions. For most research papers, though, the results section begins with a description of the study population, its demographic characteristics, the number of subjects who began the study, and the number who were excluded or were not included in the research because they withdrew or were lost in the follow-up. If there were subgroups, the demographic characteristics of each group should be presented in the beginning of the results. With extensive demographic data, a table is helpful to summarize this information. When the results section begins with the report of the demographic data, the author should be careful not to replicate the information provided earlier in the methods section.

Present Main Findings First

After describing the subjects, the author presents the main findings, followed by other findings. The order used to present this information should be consistent with the organization of the introduction and the way the purposes, questions, or hypotheses were listed earlier in the paper. This makes it easy for readers to relate the findings to the original questions for the study.

If there were subgroups in the study, the main findings should be reported first, followed by the data and related analyses for the subgroups. Along the same line, if varied outcomes measures were used, the most important outcomes should be addressed first.

Use Subheadings

Subheadings in the results section clarify the relationship of the findings to each question. This is particularly important when the results are complex and extensive. If the section is short, though, subheadings are not necessary.

A good example of using subheadings that help the reader organize the findings is from the research report by Gaston-Johansson, Ohly, Fall-Dickson. Nanda, and Kennedy (2000). The results of this study are found in Display 6.10. The subheadings used to organize the findings are consistent with the purpose, literature review, and methods, which were shown in earlier tables (See Displays 6.3 and 6.7).

Be Accurate and Precise

Researchers need to be accurate in conducting the research and reporting the findings, and the author must be careful that the writing conveys the true results. Missing information may suggest different findings to readers. Although some evidence may support the hypotheses, other data may not. The author is responsible for presenting all of the data and discussing any conflicting evidence in the discussion section of the manuscript. Data presented in the text should be consistent with the tables and figures.

Scholarly writing requires accuracy. The author accurately represents the existing knowledge about a topic, uses methods correctly, reports findings consistent with the data, and relates new information to prior research (Hegyvary, 2000). Accuracy is essential in carrying out the research and in presenting the results.

The author also should be precise in reporting the data. Rather than indicating that the data showed "promising trends in the directions hypothesized," or that the findings "tended to support the model," the author should state the exact findings of the study. Huth (1999) cautioned authors about hiding the meanings of the results behind phrases such as these (p. 71).

Report Data With Related Analyses

The data and the related statistical analyses are reported together. When reporting the mean and other descriptive statistics, the author includes the standard deviations; for inferential statistics, the value of the test, degrees of freedom, probability level, and direction of the effect are cited (APA, 1994, p. 15). The author always should check a manual of style if unsure what information to include when reporting statistics in the paper. Two helpful style manuals are the *Publication Manual of the American Psychological Association* and the *American Medical Association Manual of Style*. Both of these references provide numerous examples of how to report statistics in a manuscript.

Many authors type their own manuscripts. While most statistical symbols are printed in italics in the published article, in the manuscript the statistical symbols are underlined, not typed in italics. For example, the symbols $\underline{N}$, $\underline{M}$, and $\underline{P}$ are set in standard type and underlined in the manuscript copy, but when the article is published, these symbols will be in italic type (M, P). Greek letters, though, such as α (alpha) and β (beta) use standard type, not italics, so they should not be underlined in the manuscript. Appendix 1 lists statistical abbreviations and symbols, including how they should be typed in the manuscript and how they are then set by the publisher.

Other points should be noted when reporting statistics in the results of research papers. When citing a statistic in the narrative, the statistical term is used, not the symbol. For example, "The M score was 25" should be written as "The mean score was 25." Also remember in preparing the manuscript that an upper case N refers to the total sample, whereas a lower case n refers to a part of the sample. The actual P value should be reported (eg, $P = .04$) rather than $P < .05$ or $P < .01$, unless $P < .001$. In that case, it should be reported as $P < .001$ (AMA, 1998; Byrne, 1998). P values should not be listed as not significant (NS) since for meta-analysis, the actual value is needed (AMA, 1998).

Develop Tables for Numerical Data

Tables are an effective way of presenting detailed and complex information succinctly and clearly. In the text, the author can present the main findings and then use a table to display specific data that supplements the statements in the text. Tables support the text and therefore should not duplicate that information. For intervention studies, tables are particularly valuable in comparing groups and how differences across groups were analyzed.

As an example of how tables are useful in presenting the results, consider the need to report demographic data. Including this information in the text would require a large amount of space, would be cumbersome to report, and would be unlikely to maintain reader interest. For example, the author may want to report the number and percentage of subjects who completed education at each of these levels:

1. Less than 12th grade
2. High school graduate
3. Some college
4. College graduate (bachelor's or other 4-year degree)
5. Postgraduate or professional program (eg, master's degree, law degree).

Data such as these can be reported more efficiently in the form of a table.

Tables and figures, which are graphs, charts, diagrams, and other illustrations, have the advantage of allowing readers to visualize trends and patterns in the data more easily than when written in the narrative. Figures are particularly useful to show trends, make general comparisons, and help readers understand complex data.

Tables and figures are expensive to produce in a publication and should be used wisely by authors. Many journals limit the number, often to three, of tables and figures submitted with a manuscript. Whereas tables are valuable for presenting the findings of a study, they should not be used if the data can be presented more easily in the text.

Regarding placement in the manuscript, tables and figures follow the references, with tables first, then figures. Chapter 11 explains how to develop tables, figures, and other illustrations and provides examples of how to best design a table and figure and use them in a manuscript.

Do Not Report Individual Scores

In the results section, the author should not include the scores of individual participants or the raw data (Pyrczak & Bruce, 2000). Instead, summary statistics such as the mean and standard deviation are reported.

Discussion

The discussion section provides an opportunity to interpret the results and explain what the findings mean in relation to the purpose of the study (Display 6.11). In the discussion, the author begins by stating the main conclusion that can be drawn from the results presented earlier (Huth, 1999).

In presenting this conclusion, the author discusses whether it is consistent with prior research. Although it may be tempting to cite only studies that support the findings of the current research, it is equally important to report studies with different conclusions. In those cases, the discussion includes potential reasons for differences in findings. Perhaps there were varied subjects or settings, the instruments and measures may have differed, or the data may have been analyzed using different statistical methods. The responsibility of the author is to evaluate possible reasons for these conflicting findings.

DISPLAY 6.11	Sample Discussion

DISCUSSION

The sample characteristics describe a demographically homogeneous group of patients with breast cancer who were representative of patients awaiting autotransplantation at this comprehensive cancer center. The low-grade pain intensity and pain locations chosen (eg, chest, shoulder, and arm) and the pain descriptors (eg, dull, sore, and aching) may be related to numerous factors: previous breast cancer surgery (lumpectomy or mastectomy), a previously placed or removed central venous catheter used for the prior chemotherapy, or insufficient rehabilitation of the affected areas. Note that patients in this sample experienced pain before any invasive procedures related to the scheduled autotransplantation (eg, central line placement, bone marrow aspiration) were performed. The vaginal pain experienced also is interesting. This may be related to chemotherapy-induced mucositis or atrophic vaginitis. The continuous nature of low-intensity pain can be tiring and debilitating for patients.

Psychological distress was evident through the reporting of mild to severe depression and state anxiety. This fact demonstrates the necessity of screening for anxiety and depression in this population before admission for the autotransplantation. Most subjects chose positive coping strategies to cope with pain. Preadmission data are important as potential prognosticators of long-term quality of life (Gaston-Johansson & Foxall, 1996) and future neurobehavioral disorders (Meyers et al., 1994). Assessing patients' anxiety and depression during the preadmission period is of paramount importance to provide appropriate interventions because patients undergoing autotransplantation must adhere to the strict treatment protocol schedule.

Selected part of discussion from Gaston-Johansson, F., Ohly, K.V., Fall-Dickson, J.M., Nanda, J.P., & Kennedy, M.J. (2000). Pain, psychological distress, health status, and coping in patients with breast cancer scheduled for autotransplantation. *Oncology Nursing Forum, 26,* 1343. Adapted by permission of Oncology Nursing Society.

The discussion also allows the researcher to present implications of the study for clinical practice, teaching, or administration. What do these findings mean in terms of nursing practice? How can readers use this information in their work in nursing? Some journals have a separate section that discusses the implications of the research for practice.

It is important, though, to avoid overstating the implications. The author should avoid unqualified statements and conclusions that are not completely supported by the data, such as making comments about economic and cost benefits when these were not part of the research (ICMJE, 1997).

The author should clarify for readers if the findings can be generalized to other populations and settings. Are the findings applicable to any patient population or only ones similar to the subjects in the research? If a study was conducted with acutely ill adults in a hospital setting, the findings may have limited implications for healthy adults; research on teaching methods for use with basic students may not be applicable to teaching graduate students or staff. Many other examples could be cited. Although the implications are an important part of the discussion, they need to be based on the results of the study, considering its methods and limitations.

Limitations of the research should be addressed along with needs for further study. It is useful to suggest how the research should be extended.

Many research papers end with the discussion section, but the author may choose to include a short summary paragraph at the end highlighting major findings and what they mean for readers. This can be labeled "conclusions."

OTHER PARTS OF RESEARCH PAPER

For some research papers, the author includes an acknowledgment section to recognize the support of others in the research and preparing the manuscript. Every research paper—and most other written manuscripts—has a reference list. This is an important section in a research paper because it represents the literature used to establish why the study was conducted and its importance; a good reference list provides the critical work done previously on the topic.

Acknowledgments

For funded research, the acknowledgment specifies the financial and material support provided for the project (see Chapter 3). When an acknowledgment is included, it is placed between the text and references.

References

As discussed in Chapter 5, on reviewing and reporting the literature, the references should be current except for classic works, which may be cited in the

DISPLAY 6.12	**Order of Sections of Research Manuscript**

- Cover letter
- Copyright transfer page (if submitted with manuscript)
- Title page (numbered as page 1)
- Abstract (and key words if requested by journal)
- Text
  Introduction
  Methods
  Results
  Discussion
- Acknowledgment
- References
- Tables (with titles and footnotes)
- Figures (with legends)

paper, and should be primary rather than secondary sources. The reference list is not exhaustive but instead represents the most important work on the topic.

The format for reference lists varies with the journal. The information for authors page indicates the format to use for the journal and usually contains examples of preparing different types of references. When unsure, the author should refer to the manual of style used for that journal. Varied reference formats are discussed in Chapter 10 with examples of common ones that the author might use when writing for nursing and health care journals.

The reference list should be consistent with the references cited in the paper. All citations in the text should be on the reference list, and every reference on this list should be cited in the paper. With APA format, the author should check that the names and years of publication cited in the manuscript are the same as on the reference list. With numbered references, the author should check that the number cited in paper correctly matches the corresponding publication on the reference list.

Display 6.12 provides a summary of the parts of the research manuscript discussed in this chapter and their order. Not every manuscript, however, has each of these sections, but the order is consistent across journals. Use Display 6.12 as a checklist when submitting a research paper.

WRITING QUALITATIVE RESEARCH MANUSCRIPTS

The IMRAD format may be used as a structure for organizing qualitative research papers similar to quantitative studies. With this format, the author begins with an introduction to the study, establishing its need and importance.

Pyrczak and Bruce (2000) suggest discussing why a qualitative method was used for the study. Other sections of the manuscript are methods, which include the setting, participants, procedures, and how data were collected and analyzed; results; and discussion. These components can be seen in the abstracts of qualitative studies in Display 6.1.

Sayre (2000), in her article on the development of a grounded theory about individuals' perceptions of being a psychiatric patient, used this format to organize the research report. In the introduction, she established the lack of research on the perceptions of psychiatric patients, their explanations for being hospitalized for mental illness, and the relevance of learning more about this for clinical practice. The second section of the paper was methods. Here, Sayre described the central question for the inquiry, sample, procedures, and measures. Under the measures section, she presented how and when interviews were conducted, other data collection methods such as participant observation and review of medical records, and data analysis consistent with grounded theory methods. In the next section, she presented the findings followed by discussion. The discussion section included implications for research and clinical practice. This example illustrates how the conventional format for reporting research may be used with qualitative papers, although differences are apparent in the methods and how the findings are presented.

Presenting Findings of Qualitative Studies

Sandelowski (1998) emphasized that there is no one style for presenting qualitative research findings; the format necessarily depends on the purpose of the research, methods, and data. This is an important difference between writing quantitative and qualitative research manuscripts. When presenting the results of quantitative studies, the findings and related discussion are organized according to the purposes, questions, or hypotheses. In a qualitative research report, however, the purpose of the study, qualitative method used, and the data determine how the findings are presented.

In a qualitative research study by Redmond and Sorrell (1999) on patient satisfaction, three themes were identified in the data: knowledgeable watchfulness, thoughtful presence, and the hospital as a home away from home. In the article, the researchers provide examples of narratives that support each theme. The theme, "thoughtful presence," reflects stories shared about nurses who were present for patients in meaningful ways. The following is one narrative supporting this theme:

> Some of the nurses, I don't remember having to call them...[were] always in my room, seeing if there was anything I needed. I never had to call them. They were so caring. It was like I had friends with me, staying in the hospital (p. 70).

In this paper, the objective of the authors was to describe the views of patients in their own voices. However, with a grounded theory method, in which the goal is to discover theoretical explanations about particular phenomena (Streubert & Carpenter, 1999), the data would be used in the paper to demonstrate how a theory of patient satisfaction was developed from the interviews.

In presenting the findings of qualitative studies, the first step is to determine the central idea or point to be made from the wealth of data collected. Qualitative researchers select "which story to tell" in the manuscript from the many contained in their data set (Sandelowski, 1998). Abbott and Sapsford (1998) commented that there is more "leeway to tell the story" in a qualitative manuscript, but authors still need to demonstrate that they used a valid way of studying the problem and interpreting the data.

Organizing Qualitative Research

Data from qualitative research may be organized in the paper according to these formats: (1) by time, whereby the findings are organized as they happened to the participants, or by what the researchers themselves found about the phenomenon at different points in time; (2) by prevalence, in which the most frequently occurring themes are presented first; and (3) by using sensitizing concepts from that theory, which would be used to develop or test a theory (Sandelowski, 1998).

In reporting the data, the perspectives of the participants should be apparent to readers instead of the researcher's point of view. One way of accomplishing this is to use the conventional form of research reports in which the participants' views, the data, are presented in the results and the researcher's analysis and discussion of them are presented in the discussion section. Streubert and Carpenter (1999) emphasized the importance of writing so that readers appreciate the "richness of the data" (p. 312).

Qualitative research generates a lot of data that must be synthesized for readers. For some studies, multiple manuscripts might be written, and this decision should be made before the first manuscript is prepared. The author may have conducted a study on what it is like to care for a child with a chronic illness and the effect on the family. One manuscript might present the experiences from the parents' point of view and a second on how children cope with a chronic illness.

The decision on the journal for submission of the manuscript also influences its preparation. When writing the research paper for a clinical journal, the findings of the study and their implications for practice would be emphasized. Less attention would be given to the qualitative method and analysis of the data.

MOVING FROM THESIS AND DISSERTATION TO MANUSCRIPT

A thesis and dissertation cannot be "cut and pasted" as a manuscript; they need to be rewritten as such. A common reason for manuscript rejection is they "read like a thesis," often containing long and extensive literature reviews, which is a clue to editors and reviewers that this was a research project completed as a student (Johnson, 1996). Even experienced researchers may find it difficult to move from a research grant to a manuscript.

Often, manuscripts developed from theses and dissertations have long literature reviews, extensive reference lists, and limited relevance to the audience of the journal to which submitted. They also may extend well beyond the page limits and may contain too many tables and figures. For a clinical journal, there should be a strong discussion on the implications of the research for practice, but these manuscripts may have no implications for practice (Johnson, 1996).

What can be done to prepare a manuscript from a student research project so that it has a good chance of acceptance rather than a good chance of rejection? First, the author must decide what is the focus of the manuscript. Is the goal to present the research study, to describe the clinical implications of the research, or both? If more than one paper might be written, then the author also must decide how many and what types of manuscripts to prepare. Second, the author needs to choose a journal that would provide an avenue for publishing the intended manuscript. Clinical journals want manuscripts with practice implications. Research journals want manuscripts that describe the study methods and findings, even if implications also are discussed. Third, think about the target audience so that the manuscript is geared to the readers of the journal.

Once these preliminary decisions are made, the next steps involve adapting the research project to a manuscript format. Some techniques follow:

- Shorten the title if needed.
- Develop a new outline that reflects the format of the journal.
- Write new subheadings to reflect the goals of the manuscript rather than using the subheadings required for the thesis or dissertation.
- Shorten the background of the study and introduce the purpose of manuscript early in the introduction.
- Synthesize the literature review, present the most important studies, and consider integrating the literature within the introduction (depending on the journal's format).
- Review sample research articles in the journal to determine if they include a separate section on the theoretical framework. If not, integrate a brief statement of the framework in the literature review. If

articles include a section for the theoretical framework, shorten the one from the thesis and describe it briefly in the manuscript.

- Shorten the methods section, omit the rationale for the methods, and shorten the discussion of psychometric properties of the measures unless submitting the manuscript to a research journal.
- Revise the description of the sample and presentation of the demographic data to fit the journal being considered for submission.
- Watch the extent of statistical analysis described in the manuscript and write for the audience.
- If submitting to a clinical journal, emphasize practice implications.
- Shorten the reference list.
- Include only essential tables and figures up to a maximum of three.
- Rewrite the manuscript to make it consistent with the writing style of the journal and appropriate for its readers, who need the information.
- Plan the manuscript wisely considering page limits, which are typically 15 to 18 pages of text.

 ## SUMMARY

Nursing research is of little value if the findings are not made available for use by clinicians and others who need the research results for their work. Nurses who conduct research are responsible for reporting the results in journals that are read by nurses who can use the information in their practice, teaching, or management. By publishing the findings of research, nurses advance the body of knowledge of nursing and contribute to the scientific basis of nursing practice. Communicating the findings of research promotes the critique and replication of studies and is essential for research utilization in nursing. Nurses also need research data to establish evidence for their decisions and interventions.

The conventional format for writing research papers is the IMRAD format—introduction, methods, results and discussion—or an adaptation of this, depending on the journal and type of research. IMRAD provides a way of organizing the paper and specifies in advance the headings for it.

The first section of the manuscript is the introduction, which is the author's opportunity to explain the nature and background of the study, its purpose, and its importance. The author begins the introduction with a discussion of the specific problem addressed by the research and its significance. This discussion provides a framework for reading the related literature; determining how the study builds on previous research on the topic; and understanding the relationship of the purposes, questions, or hypotheses to the problem.

The literature review describes what is already known about the topic and what needs to be studied, thereby justifying the current project. Gaps in knowledge and limitations of prior studies are emphasized to provide support for the study. The literature review may be incorporated into the introduction or presented as a separate section in the manuscript. The literature review may contain the discussion of the conceptual or theoretical framework that guided the study, or the framework may be included in a separate section.

The last part of the introduction includes the purposes of the study, questions the research was designed to answer, or hypotheses that were tested. There are differences in how the introductions are written in nursing journals, so the author should review sample articles before beginning the manuscript.

The next section of the manuscript is methods. In this section, information is presented about the study design, subjects, measures, procedures, and data analysis in that order.

In the results section, the author presents the findings of the study. The findings should answer each of the research questions and address the original purposes of the study. Here, the author presents the data and its analysis but without discussion of the findings.

The discussion section provides an opportunity to interpret the results and explain what the findings mean. In the discussion, the author begins by stating the main conclusion that can be drawn from the results. The discussion allows the researcher to present implications of the study for clinical practice, teaching, or administration. Limitations of the research should be addressed, along with needs for further study.

The IMRAD format also may be used as a broad structure for organizing qualitative research papers. With this format, the author begins with an introduction to the study, establishing its need and importance. Other sections of the manuscript are methods, which include the setting, participants, procedures, and how data were collected and analyzed; results; and discussion. The content in each section, however, reflects the purpose of the study, qualitative method, and data.

A thesis and dissertation need to be rewritten as a manuscript; they cannot be used as is. Often, manuscripts developed from theses and dissertations are too long and are not relevant for the journal to which they are submitted. Strategies for preparing a manuscript from a thesis and dissertation are detailed in the chapter.

REFERENCES

Abbott, P., & Sapsford, R. (1998). *Research methods for nurses and the caring professions* (2nd ed.). Philadelphia: Open University Press.

American Medical Association. (1998). *Manual of style: A guide for authors and editors* (9th ed.). Baltimore: Lippincott Williams & Wilkins.

American Psychological Association (APA). (1994). *Publication manual of the American Psychological Association* (4th ed.). Washington, DC: APA.

Antle, D.E. (2000). Ensuring competency in nurse repositioning of the pulmonary artery catheter. *Dimensions of Critical Care Nursing, 19*(2), 44–51.

Brown, S.T. (2000). Outcomes analysis of a pain management project for two rural hospitals. *Journal of Nursing Care Quality, 14*(4), 28–34.

Byrne, D.W. (1998). Publishing your medical research paper. Baltimore: Lippincott Williams & Wilkins.

Gaston-Johansson, F., Ohly, K.V., Fall-Dickson, J.M., Nanda, J.P., & Kennedy, M.J. (2000). Pain, psychological distress, health status, and coping in patients with breast cancer scheduled for autotransplantation. *Oncology Nursing Forum, 26*, 1337–1345.

Hegyvary, S.T. (2000). Standards of scholarly writing. *Journal of Nursing Scholarship, 32*, 112.

Hicks, C. (1995). The shortfall in published research: A study of nurses' research and publication activities. *Journal of Advanced Nursing, 21*, 594–604.

Huth, E.J. (1999). *Writing and publishing in medicine* (3rd ed.). Baltimore: Lippincott Williams & Wilkins.

International Committee of Medical Journal Editors. (1997). Uniform requirements for manuscripts submitted to biomedical journals. *Annals of Internal Medicine, 126*(1), 36–47. [On-line]. Also available: *http://www.icmje.org/*.

Johnson, S.H. (1996). Adapting a thesis to publication style: Meeting editors' expectations. *Dimensions of Critical Care Nursing, 15*, 160–167.

Lyder, C. (1999). Interpreting and reporting research findings. In J.A. Fain (Ed.), *Reading, understanding, and applying nursing research* (pp. 229–244). Philadelphia: F.A. Davis.

MacLean, S.L. (1999). Writing the research report. In M.A. Mateo, & K.T. Kirchhoff (Eds.), *Using and conducting nursing research in the clinical setting* (2nd ed., pp. 328–338). Philadelphia: W.B. Saunders.

McPheeters, M., & Lohr, K.N. (1999). Evidence-based practice and nursing: Commentary. *Outcomes Management for Nursing Practice, 3*, 99–101.

National Library of Medicine. (2000). ELHILL MEDLINE data element descriptions and other information. [On-line]. Available: *http://www.nlm.nih.gov/databases/license/medlars_elements2.html#ab*. Accessed July 20, 2000.

Nesbitt, B.J., & Heidrich, S.M. (2000). Sense of coherence and illness appraisal in older women's quality of life. *Research in Nursing and Health, 23*, 25–34.

Nicoll, L.H., & Beyea, S.C. (1999). Research utilization. In J.A. Fain (Ed.), *Reading, understanding, and applying nursing research* (pp. 261–280). Philadelphia: F.A. Davis.

Oermann, M.H., & Templin, T. (2000). Important attributes of quality health care: Consumer perspectives. *Journal of Nursing Scholarship, 32*, 167–172.

Paul, S. (2000). Impact of a nurse-managed heart failure clinic: A pilot study. *American Journal of Critical Care, 9*, 140–146.

Polit, D.F., & Hungler, B.P. (1997). *Essentials of nursing research: Methods, appraisal, and utilization* (4th ed.). Philadelphia: Lippincott-Raven.

Pyrczak, F., & Bruce, R.R. (2000). *Writing empirical research reports* (3rd ed.). Los Angeles: Pyrczak Publishing.

Redmond, G.M., & Sorrell, J.M. (1999). Studying patient satisfaction: Patient voices of quality. *Outcomes Management for Nursing Practice, 3,* 67–72.

Rosswurm, M.A., & Larrabee, J.H. (1999). A model for change to evidence-based practice. *Image: Journal of Nursing Scholarship, 31,* 317–322.

Sandelowski, M. (1998). Writing a good read: Strategies for re-presenting qualitative data. *Research in Nursing and Health, 21,* 375–382.

Sayre, J. (2000). The patient's diagnosis: Explanatory models of mental illness. *Qualitative Health Research, 10*(1), 71–83.

Streubert, H.J., & Carpenter, D.R. (1999). *Qualitative research in nursing* (2nd ed.). Philadelphia: Lippincott Williams & Wilkins.

Tornquist, E., & Funk, S.G. (1993). How to report research with clarity, coherence, and grace. *Journal of Emergency Nursing, 19,* 498–502.

Winland-Brown, J.E., & Valiante, J. (2000). Effectiveness of different medication management approaches on elders' medication adherence. *Outcomes Management for Nursing Practice, 4,* 172–176.

CLINICAL PRACTICE ARTICLES AND OTHER TYPES OF WRITING

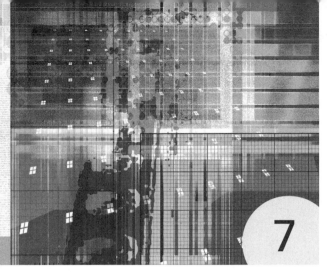

7

This chapter presents strategies for writing clinical practice, professional role, issue, philosophical and theoretical, and review articles. Other forms of writing such as case reports, editorials, book reviews, letters to the editor, and articles for consumer and nonprofessional audiences also are examined. These types of manuscripts differ in their intended purpose, their format, and, often, writing style. The last section of the chapter provides guidelines for writing chapters and books.

CLINICAL PRACTICE ARTICLES

Many nursing journals address topics in clinical practice. These articles disseminate new knowledge and skills for patient care, enabling nurses to stay current in clinical practice. With this type of article, nurses in one setting can describe their practice innovations for use and testing by nurses in other settings. They can discuss issues faced in patient care and how they resolved those issues, and they can share nursing measures that worked and ones that did not work, so that nurses can build on the experiences of others rather than starting from the beginning. Otherwise, the benefits of nurses' clinical experiences are confined only to their patients and colleagues working with them (Ashworth, 1998). To remain competent, professionals need to continually expand their knowledge base and skills; clinical practice articles provide a source of information to meet this need.

Idea for Clinical Article

The process for writing a clinical article begins with an idea. This idea may come from the author's experience with a patient, a clinical situation involving the author, the author's projects or activities in the clinical setting, or from a discussion with nursing staff and other providers. The idea for a manuscript may result from a frustrating experience encountered by the author or an issue that the author faced in practice and eventually resolved. Clinical articles often result from the nurse's own experiences with patients, families, and staff and, later, a reflection on those experiences. Thus, one primary source of ideas for clinical articles is the author's own clinical practice and interactions with nurses.

Another source of ideas for clinical articles is from lectures and presentations. Educators in academic and clinical settings are continually preparing lectures and other presentations, many of which pertain to clinical practice or are intended to keep nurses up to date. If the lecture deals with new interventions for patient care, a change in practice that will benefit patients across clinical settings, a trend in nursing and health care, or an issue involving patients and consumers, these lectures may be rewritten as manuscripts. Lectures and other types of presentations provide the basis for publications in general or specialized clinical journals, depending on the topic.

Ideas for clinical articles also may evolve from research studies, literature reviews, educational experiences, and other activities that lead to new information or a different perspective about nursing practice. Presenting new information for readers is critical: many manuscripts are rejected because the content is not new and has been reported before (Fondiller, 1994).

When deciding whether the idea is worth pursuing for a clinical article, the author should answer these questions:

- Is the idea new and innovative?
- If the idea is not new, does it provide a different perspective to current practice?
- Is the content clinically relevant and applicable to nursing practice in a specialty area or in general?
- Do nurses *need* this information for their practice and will it improve patient care?
- Will the information be valuable in keeping nurses up to date about trends in nursing and health care?
- Will the content inform readers about the types of activities and work that nurses are doing in other settings and places?

These questions give authors a framework for deciding if the clinical topic is worth pursuing for publication.

Purpose of Article

From this idea, the author specifies the purpose of the manuscript. This is an important step because clinical articles can have many different perspectives. What is the goal of the paper? Is it to present new nursing practices and patient care or provide a different perspective to an accepted practice? Will scientific rationale and related research be emphasized? Is the intent to describe nursing interventions and their effectiveness, to present a clinical pathway and how well it worked with a specific patient population, or to describe an interdisciplinary plan of care? Answering questions such as these enables the author to clarify the purpose of the paper.

Intended Readers

The next step is to identify the intended readers of the manuscript. These readers may be staff nurses, advanced practice nurses, and nurse managers. Who will read the article dictates the content included in it.

Clinical articles may be written for a general nursing audience, providing information to help nurses in different specialties and settings to stay current. Other clinical articles address nurses who practice in a particular clinical area. These articles focus on specific patient populations and health problems. This is an important difference when deciding on the journal for submission because it determines the complexity of the content and types of examples used in the discussion. Clinical articles written for a general nursing audience describe the content more broadly and use common examples. The content may not be appropriate for a specialty journal because those nurses already may be familiar with it.

In planning the content, the author takes into consideration the knowledge and background of the intended readers. Knowing the journal's audience also guides the author in selecting terms and examples consistent with the background of readers (Stepanski, 1999). Display 2.1 provides a list of questions for authors to use in clarifying the intended audience of the paper.

In preparing the manuscript, the author also determines what prerequisite knowledge readers need to understand the content. This guides the author in deciding on background material to include in the paper so that new information is clear. For example, in preparing a manuscript on a new treatment for burns for the journal *Dermatology Nursing*, limited background information would be needed about evaluating and managing burn wounds. However, if the manuscript is written for nurses across specialties to update them and for general interest, more discussion would be required about types of burns, evaluating burn wounds, current practices in caring for patients with burns, and how this new treatment differs. Expanded discussion on scientific rationale also might be needed.

Format of Clinical Practice Articles

The format for writing clinical articles depends on the purpose of the article and the journal for submission. Some journals have departments for different types of clinical articles. The author decides before beginning the paper if it will be developed for a department in a journal because these manuscripts often are shorter and more focused than the main articles.

There is no standard format for writing clinical articles. A manuscript that presents nursing interventions for patients with a particular health problem will be organized differently than one that reviews pharmacology. In contrast to research articles, which follow a standard format, clinical manuscripts vary because of the wide range of topics addressed in them.

Some general guidelines for writing clinical articles follow. However, these guidelines may not pertain to every manuscript, depending on its focus.

Title

Every clinical paper needs a title. The title informs readers about the new information presented in the paper. Key words that represent the content should be used in the title, and the title should be concise.

Nurses are busy professionals, and with a series of articles to read in a journal and limited time, the title needs to draw the attention of readers. For example, *"No More Surprises:* Screening Patients for Alcohol Abuse" is more of an attention-getter than the title, "*Assessment* of Patients for Alcohol Abuse."

Similar to research articles, one title may be written, or it may be developed with a subtitle that provides more specific information about the paper. When subtitles are used, the terms that represent the main focus of the article should be placed first in the title:

- Single title: "Nursing Care After Pneumonectomy in Patients With Invasive Pulmonary Aspergillosis" (McHale & Barth, 2000)
- Title with subtitle: "Patients With Invasive Pulmonary Aspergillosis: Nursing Care After Pneumonectomy."

Abstract

Not all clinical manuscripts are submitted with an abstract, but when an abstract is required, it should concisely present the content included in the paper and its clinical implications. The abstract is the author's first chance to convince readers that the paper is important to read.

The American Psychological Association (1994) limits abstracts to 120 words, although for some journals they may be longer, up to 250 words (American Medical Association, 1998). When abstracts are required, the author guidelines indicate how to prepare them for a particular journal.

Examples of abstracts for clinical articles are given in Display 7.1. Both abstracts inform the readers about the content in the article and its practical implications for nurses.

Introduction

The first section of the manuscript is the introduction. Here, the author presents the purpose of the paper, an overview of its topics, the relevance of the content for clinical practice, and the value of the article to nurses.

The first or lead paragraph of the introduction is the most important: if it is unclear or poorly written, readers will not continue with the article. The lead-in paragraph also needs to capture reader's interest. The author can use the lead-in paragraph to indicate the purpose, topics, and relevance to clinical practice:

> Many patients are unable to report the pain they are experiencing. This places them at risk for pain that is undertreated because of communication problems. This article describes how to assess patient's pain using the basic measures of pain intensity as a framework and following six other steps. The information is important for nurses when caring for patients who are unable to report their pain.

DISPLAY 7.1   **Sample Abstracts for Clinical Articles**

EXAMPLE 1

Neck masses often present a diagnostic challenge to the primary care provider. Etiologies range from benign inflammations to life-threatening malignancies. Placing the etiologies into three broad categories is helpful when considering the extensive differential diagnosis for a neck mass: congenital, inflammatory/infectious, and neoplastic. This article discusses the evaluation and subsequent determination of whether a neck mass is significant and warrants further evaluation or is insignificant and simply may be observed. By performing a thorough history and physical examination, primary care providers can narrow the possibilities, differentiate between significant and insignificant neck masses, and select the appropriate treatment.[1]

EXAMPLE 2

The variety of available chest drainage systems makes it more important than ever for nurses to understand what is out there and how these systems work. Nurses are responsible for managing chest drains and need to know which drain is best suited for which situation.[2]

[1]From Prisco, M.K. (2000). Evaluating neck masses. *The Nurse Practitioner, 25*(4), 30. Reprinted by permission of Springhouse, © 2000 Springhouse Corporation/*www.springnet.com*.
[2]From Carroll, P. (2000). Exploring chest drain options. *RN, 63*(10), 50. © 2000 Medical Economics, Montvale, NJ. Reprinted by permission.

Other types of lead-in paragraphs introduce the topic but focus more on getting the readers' attention. Three types of opening paragraphs that focus primarily on getting the attention of the readers are anecdotal opening, placing the reader in the clinical situation, and using statistics.

Anecdotal Openings

Anecdotal openings share a real or simulated clinical experience or present a case scenario with which readers can identify professionally or personally. The opening may describe a patient and the patient's problems, may begin with a case scenario, or may describe the nurse's experiences and feelings when caring for a patient. Anecdotal openings capture readers' interest by indicating the professional or personal relevance of the information.

The following is an example of an anecdotal opening to an article on adrenal crisis, the related physiology, how to differentiate it from other conditions, nursing care and related medical management, and how to avert future episodes:

> Carol Baran, age 36, is brought to the ED at 6:15 AM. As Ms. Baran's husband leads her in, you observe her unsteady and wandering gait. She says she was awake and restless all night with chills, sweating, nausea, and abdominal pain. Yesterday, she had several episodes of vomiting; because of severe nausea, her only oral intake has been sips of water....You realize you are not dealing with a simple case of flu and immediately obtain IV access while Ms. Baran tells you her medical history. She's been taking the glucocorticoid hydrocortisone, 10 mg each morning and 5 mg each evening, since her right adrenal gland was removed because of a tumor (Carson, 2000, p. 49).

This example also shows the contrast in writing style from research articles, which are more formal and use a more scholarly style. Often, clinical journals prefer the more informal style of writing seen in the example.

Placement in Clinical Situation

A similar type of lead-in paragraph is one that places the reader in the clinical situation. In the following introduction, the nurse is involved in the scenario as a realistic participant who needs to make decisions and act in response to the situation. The question for the reader is, "What would you do in this clinical situation?" An example of this type of attention-getter is as follows:

> You have been working in the clinical agency for nearly 10 months. Recently, you noticed a colleague having difficulty completing her assignments on time. She often is late for work and asks you to cover for her. Today, you notice her moving from one patient to the next without washing her hands.

This example provides the clinical context for the article and involves the reader as a participant. Here, the reader "becomes" the nurse involved in this dilemma, which the article analyzes, providing options on which the nurse may act. A personal experience of the nurse, positive or negative, also serves to "connect with readers" who may have had similar experiences.

Use of Statistics

Another attention-getter is the use of statistics, which demonstrate the impact of the information on patient care, the nurse's own practice, or health care in general. In this type of introduction, statistics illustrate the magnitude of the problem and its implications, signifying the importance of the article:

> The next time you find yourself in a room full of adults, consider this: 1 in every 13 meets the diagnostic criteria for alcoholism and alcohol abuse—a total of 14 million Americans.[1] The numbers of teens are equally alarming: the National Council on Alcohol and Drug Dependence reports that 5.1 million Americans between the ages of 12 and 20 binge (consume five or more drinks on a single occasion) at least once a month[2] (Henderson-Martin, 2000, p. 27).

This lead-in paragraph to an article on screening patients for alcohol abuse uses alarming facts to illustrate the magnitude of the problem.

Text

The text, or body of the paper, follows the introduction and varies depending on the content. Because clinical manuscripts address a wide range of topics—from general practice updates to specific interventions for one type of patient problem—there is no one outline that can be used. Some principles, though, guide development of the text for clinical articles:

- Organize the content from simple to complex and from known to unknown.
- Provide background information and scientific rationale so that readers can understand the reasons underlying problems, interventions, and outcomes.
- Focus on what nurses need to learn about assessment of patients, the meaning of signs and symptoms, related diagnostic tests, and interpretation of data.
- Focus on what nurses need to learn about patient responses, problems, and diagnoses; interventions; and outcomes. Emphasize related research and implications for clinical practice.
- Focus on nursing management rather than medical management, even though this content also may be included in the paper. The goal is to help nurses assess patients and effectively manage their problems.

- If using a scenario as an attention-getter, relate the content in the paper to the scenario so that readers can see how this new information can be used in clinical practice.

- Use examples from clinical practice in the paper to assist readers in applying the new information to patient care. Consider using one scenario throughout the paper as a way of demonstrating how the concepts relate to assessment, diagnoses, interventions, and outcomes. In this way, the scenario provides a model of how the new information is used in clinical practice.

- Answer the following questions: "Why?" "What if...?" "What are the other options and possible decisions?" and "How?" Answering these questions promotes the nurses' critical thinking about the content.

- When using an acronym, write it out at its first mention in the paper.

- Use a writing style that is consistent with the journal. Several clinical journals use "I" and "you" rather than "the nurse." The author should gather information about writing style before beginning the draft.

- Use frequent and specific subheadings that clearly describe the content in that section. The author should review a few articles in the journal for submission because types of subheadings often vary. Some journals use more formal subheadings than others. This difference can be seen in Table 7.1.

The extent of background information to include is based on the author's professional judgment and an understanding of the reader's needs. When presenting new information not available in nursing textbooks or through other

TABLE 7.1

Comparison of Subheadings for a Clinical Article

Formal	Informal*
Deep Vein Thrombosis (DVT)	What is DVT?
Etiology	What Causes DVT?
Diagnosis	Diagnosis Is Made With Sharp Eye and Tests
Pharmacological Management	Proactive Intervention: Pharmacologic Options
Nursing Interventions	Nursing Actions Can Help
Anticoagulant Therapy	If Patient Develops Clot
Nursing Care	Getting Patient Back on His Feet

*Adapted from Breen, P. (2000). DVT: What every nurse should know. *RN, 63*(4), 58–62.

resources, the author includes more background material than would be necessary for a manuscript on a new direction in clinical practice but for a common patient problem known by most readers.

An example of this strategy is seen in an article on nursing care of patients with invasive pulmonary aspergillosis who require pneumonectomy. Because the disease is uncommon and there is limited literature available, the authors provide extensive background information so that readers understand the nursing care for these patients who present a challenge to critical care nurses. The content includes etiology, prevalence, risk factors, pathophysiologic features, clinical manifestations, diagnosis, medical and surgical treatments, and nursing care, organized in that order. The authors include a sample care plan with nursing diagnoses, interventions, and outcomes, and many examples throughout the article to illustrate how the content applies to patient care (McHale & Barth, 2000).

Conclusion

Every clinical article, similar to other papers, ends with a conclusion. The conclusion summarizes the information and its value to nurses in their own clinical practice. It also may suggest areas where further work is needed, such as testing of an intervention across settings, but the conclusion should not introduce new information. The conclusion encourages nurses to implement the interventions presented in the paper, change nursing practice, or act on the information (Black, 1996). Often, the conclusion suggests an action that the nurse—or nursing as a profession—should take, such as the need for research and legislation. The conclusion generally is one to two paragraphs long.

Many of these same principles can be used in writing other types of articles discussed in the remaining sections of the chapter. Authors should follow the format of the journal for submission and gear the paper to intended readers.

 ## PROFESSIONAL ROLE ARTICLES

Another type of manuscript relates to the professional role of the nurse. These papers are intended for nurse practitioners, clinical nurse specialists, educators, managers, administrators, and nurses in other positions. Rather than providing information applicable to patient care, the focus instead is on role development, performance, and evaluation.

In these manuscripts, the author presents content that helps readers to perform more effectively in a particular role. Articles of this nature communicate the knowledge and skills needed for carrying out a role in nursing, assist nurses in developing competencies for performing a role, address issues faced by nurses in their roles and how they resolved them, and describe trends in their practices.

Readers of *Nurse Educator*, for instance, learn about trends in program development, instructional methods for classroom and clinical teaching, evaluation strategies, and test construction—information that assists them in performing their role as a teacher. In the *Journal of Nursing Administration* (JONA), articles provide information for top-level nurse executives and their immediate associates on developments and advances in leadership in patient care nursing, and on tools to function in their roles in the changing health care system (JONA, 2000).

Clinical Nurse Specialist addresses the role of the advanced practice nurse as researcher, consultant, clinician, peer, and patient educator, regardless of specialty (Clinical Nurse Specialist, 2000). The mission of *The Nurse Practitioner: The American Journal of Primary Health Care* (NPJ) is to provide clinical and professional information to meet the needs of nurse practitioners and other advanced practice nurses. Although many of the articles focus on the management of acute and chronic illnesses, the journal publishes articles on issues that affect nurse practitioners and ways to advance their role (NPJ, 2000).

 PROFESSIONAL ISSUES ARTICLES

What about issues in nursing? Information about trends and issues in nursing is becoming increasingly available on the Internet, but nurses need publications that analyze issues, why and how they developed, varied positions that can be taken, and multiple strategies for resolving them. Many clinical journals publish this type of paper. Some journals have a department or column on professional issues affecting nurses in that area of clinical practice, societal issues facing patients, and other opinion pieces. The *Online Journal of Issues in Nursing* (OJIN) presents a variety of perspectives on issues in nursing across clinical specialties and settings. The journal recognizes that individuals have differing views on issues and provides a forum for readers to express their opinions and understand others' views (OJIN, 2000).

These papers can begin with a discussion of the issue and why and how it developed. Some papers address information needed to understand the issue itself, increasing nurses' knowledge about it. In these manuscripts, the goal is to improve understanding of issues in health care and nursing practice, not for nurses to assume a position about an issue. For example, a paper might provide an overview of prenatal testing, a historical perspective, examples of prenatal tests, nursing views, and ethical considerations. Rather than taking a position about prenatal testing, the goal of the author is to present information about the issue and a foundation to better understand related ethical decisions.

In another approach, the author analyzes the issue from different points of view. In this type of paper, the issue and the varied perspectives possible are presented for readers with a rationale. For example, a paper on whether continuing education should be mandatory or voluntary might present both positions and the rationale for each, leaving the readers to decide on their position. Alternatively, the author might take one point of view and present a rationale to support it. For example, the author might develop a paper on why continuing education should be mandatory rather than voluntary.

With issue papers, the author includes the assumptions on which thinking is based, the evidence used to guide the analysis of the issue, and how the author's own position was developed. In preparing these manuscripts, the author is advised to be clear about personal biases and perspectives so that the content reflects an objective analysis of the issue rather than the author's view only.

 ## PHILOSOPHICAL AND THEORETICAL ARTICLES

Other topics are philosophical or deal with theory development or testing. The format used to develop these manuscripts relates to the goals of the paper, philosophical theory used for its development or the position taken, or structure of the theory or framework.

Manuscripts of this type might discuss the development of nursing theory, present the results of the testing of concepts and theories, analyze an existing theory and propose an extension of it or an alternative theory, and compare different theories. Varied philosophical perspectives can be analyzed and compared. In general, these papers should include a review of the literature that serves as the foundation for the author's thinking and perspective. In writing philosophical and theoretical manuscripts, the author should be careful with how ideas are presented and ordered so that they are logical and placed in the appropriate sequence. A sound argument must be presented to support ideas and defend them using theory and research.

As an example, Sanford (2000) developed a nursing perspective for patient education based on a conceptualization of caring. She began the paper by describing the philosophical tenets on which the theory was based, including the philosophy of nursing and of patient education. Next, she presented the assumptions derived from these philosophies that served as the premise for the theory. Using recommendations from the literature on middle-range theory development, Sanford organized the rest of the content according to these recommendations. Therefore, the content and its organization reflect concepts of theory development in nursing.

Some journals in nursing are devoted to nursing science and theory development. For example, the primary purposes of *Advances in Nursing Science* (ANS) are to contribute to the development of nursing science and to promote the application of theories and research findings to nursing practice. Articles deal with theory development, concept analysis, practical application of research and theory, and other areas related to nursing science (ANS, 2000). *Nursing Science Quarterly* (NSQ) publishes manuscripts focusing on nursing theory development, theory-based nursing practice, and quantitative and qualitative research related to existing nursing frameworks (NSQ, 2000).

INTEGRATIVE REVIEW AND META-ANALYSIS ARTICLES

The results of integrative reviews and meta-analyses also may be prepared for publication. The goal of an integrative review is to identify studies that address a research question, evaluate them, interpret results, and suggest implications for practice. A meta-analysis extends the critique of the research articles to include statistical analysis of the outcomes of similar studies (Beyea & Nicoll, 1998).

Integrative Review Articles

For an integrative review article, the author identifies past research on a particular topic, critiques these studies, and then draws conclusions about the findings. The review of the literature is guided by a research question or problem to be solved. The review article is not a summary of each study found on a topic; studies are critiqued and findings are integrated.

Need for Integrative Review Articles

Integrative review articles are important because they provide evidence for making decisions about clinical practice. Rosswurm and Larrabee (1999) developed a model for evidence-based practice that includes six steps: (1) assess the need for a change in practice, (2) link the problems with interventions and outcomes using standardized classifications, (3) synthesize the best evidence, (4) design practice changes, (5) implement and evaluate the changes in practice, and (6) integrate and maintain them. In step 3, the literature is reviewed critically, and practitioners evaluate the strengths and weaknesses of each study, identify gaps in knowledge, and rate the quality of the evidence. In this process, the literature is synthesized as a basis for making decisions about clinical practice or determining if more work needs to done before changes are made in practice.

An integrative review of the literature must be thorough and systematic. It should result in the development of new knowledge that can be translated into practice or should highlight areas needing further investigation (Bell, 1998). These articles communicate what is known and not yet known about dimensions of nursing such as clinical practice, teaching, and administration.

Writing an Integrative Review Article

In the introduction of an integrative review article, the author presents the background of the problem and why an analysis of the literature is needed to better understand the problem or answer the question. This gives the reader a framework for why the review was completed.

The criteria for including studies in the review, criteria for evaluating each study, and how generalizations were drawn from the research are reported in the manuscript. This information is important so that readers understand how the review was conducted.

If the literature on the topic has been analyzed previously, the author should explain why the review was repeated and how the current manuscript differs from earlier review articles. Perhaps earlier reviews included only one age group, one type of clinical setting, or patients with certain problems. It also may be that prior reviews were inconclusive or that recent research has changed what we know about the topic.

Guidelines for writing integrative review articles follow:

- In the introduction, include a discussion on the background of the problem and why the review was indicated.
- Report the questions answered in the review.
- If other reviews were done on the same topic, explain why this review is indicated and how it differs from earlier work.
- Report the methods used for the review, including the definition of the topic and how it was limited (eg, by age of patients), criteria for selecting articles for the review, bibliographic databases searched with years searched and search terms, and how quantitative data across studies were integrated.
- Use a logical sequence for reporting the results of the review. For some reviews, the nursing process may be used (Beyea & Nicoll, 1998), but in general the topic determines how the findings are organized.
- Use subheadings that clearly define how the results are organized.
- Present the evidence found to support conclusions reached and which questions remain unanswered.
- Write a strong conclusion that summarizes the major findings from the review. The conclusions should specify the implications for clinical practice, teaching, administration, or management and where further study is needed.

Meta-Analysis Articles

A meta-analysis allows the researcher to compare results across similar studies using statistical techniques. With a meta-analysis, the researcher also can examine the effects of extraneous variables—such as sample characteristics—on the results (Harrison, 1999). Meta-analyses provide strong evidence for practice, but in many areas of nursing, there is not enough available research for a meta-analysis.

Huth (1999) suggested that meta-analysis articles follow the traditional research format. The title and abstract should make it clear that the manuscript is a meta-analysis and not a report of a research study. The meta-analysis paper should be organized beginning with an introduction, followed by a description of the methods and protocol used for the analysis, presentation of the findings, and discussion. In presenting the findings, authors should focus on reporting study characteristics and exact statistical values and P levels; a summary table of basic descriptive and inferential statistics might be prepared to accompany the manuscript (Beck, 1999).

 ## CASE REPORTS

Case reports provide new information on nursing practice and the care of patients with particular health problems through the presentation of an actual case. These manuscripts often begin with why the case was selected and its importance to nursing practice, and continue with a description of the case and related care by nurses and other disciplines. For example, Jones (2000) presented a case report on managing the care of a premature infant at 29 weeks' gestation who experienced dehiscence secondary to bowel repair. The case demonstrated the effectiveness of the interventions for wound healing in this fragile population.

Although a single case study and its findings cannot be generalized, these articles can be used to describe patient care; illustrate how concepts, theories, and research are used in practice; present issues in a patient's care and strategies for resolving them; and apply new information to a real or hypothetical case. Case reports also can be used for promoting the clinical judgment, decision-making, and critical thinking skills of nurses. A case can be presented with possible decisions and different options for resolution. Consequences of each decision can be examined, followed by the decision the nurse made in the case.

A case report typically includes the following content areas:

- Introductory discussion: The introduction describes why this case is significant and how it will help nurses to better understand their patients' problems and care: An effective introduction makes it clear why the case is worth reading.

- Description of the case: In this section, relevant data about the case and background information are presented. The case presentation may follow a chronologic sequence or may represent one particular phase of the health problem.

- Nursing care: This section includes care planned and implemented for the patient, family, or community; evaluation of its effectiveness; and implications for nursing practice. Changes in practice suggested as a result of this case may be included in this section of the manuscript.

- Alternate decisions possible in the case and consequences of each: This is an important section if the case is designed to promote nurses' clinical judgment and critical thinking skills. How nurses might approach the patient's care from different perspectives also is included in this section.

- Ethical considerations: Cases may be used to present ethical issues in a patient's care and strategies for resolving ethical dilemmas.
- Conclusions with implications for clinical practice: The manuscript should conclude with a discussion of the implications of this case for the nurse's own practice and what it means to the care of other patients.

Publications in nursing, medicine, and other health care disciplines must protect the rights of individuals to privacy. Patient names, initials, and case numbers should be omitted from published case reports. The uniform requirements of the International Committee of Medical Journal Editors (ICMJE) suggest that identifying information about patients should not be published unless (1) it is essential for scientific purposes, (2) the patient or legally authorized representative gives written informed consent for publication, and (3) the patient or legally authorized representative is allowed to review the manuscript before giving informed consent for the information to be published (ICMJE, 1997). When informed consent is obtained, it should be indicated in the published article.

The author is cautioned to query the editor if interested in a case report because some journals do not publish case reports as articles. For these journals, there may be a department for which the case would be appropriate. As an example, the *Journal of Obstetric, Gynecologic, and Neonatal Nursing* (2000) has a category for manuscripts that are case reports—reviews of cases on nursing care that present new information for clinical practice.

EDITORIALS

Some journals have editorials that are written only by the journal's editor, but with other publications, nurses may be asked to write the editorial. Preparing an editorial for a journal requires a different type of writing than used for other manuscripts. Often, editorials are issue oriented, related to the theme of articles in the journal. For example, if the theme of the journal is genetic counseling, the editorial may focus on related ethical considerations.

An editorial also may be a critical review of an original paper in the journal or a summary of new developments in the field. Editorials that comment on papers in the journal may provide an alternative view of the issue or even a different interpretation of the data. New findings may have been presented recently, and readers need to be aware of them when they read the article; editorials are a way of providing these other perspectives. An editorial also might emphasize the practice implications of articles in the journal.

Editorials usually are short, so the first task of the author is to plan the content within a limited number of words. In contrast to manuscripts that generally range from 15 to 18 pages of text, editorials may be only 3 to 6 typed pages.

Many editorials can be written using the following format: statement of the problem or issue, possible solutions and approaches, supporting evidence for each, and the author's conclusion based on this evidence. In some situations, the author may indicate a lack of existing evidence to support a decision or an action, concluding that more study is needed.

 ## BOOK REVIEWS

Nurses might write book reviews for journals describing what the book is about and addressing its quality. This is a good opportunity for nurses with limited writing experience. Book reviews typically are short pieces, similar in length to editorials, and authors need to communicate their ideas clearly and succinctly.

The purpose of the review is to inform readers about the quality of the book and its content so that they can decide whether to purchase it. Johnson (1997) cautions authors to make specific comments about the book rather than unsubstantiated conclusions. For instance, rather than saying the book is "too basic for experienced nurses and they should not buy it," the author can cite examples from the book that demonstrate the depth of content and then conclude that the book is "most useful to new graduates."

The following are guidelines for writing a book review:

- Identify the purpose of the book. This generally is stated in the preface and introduction. Then assess if the book achieves this purpose.
- Describe the types of readers for whom the book would be valuable, for instance, students as a course text, inservice educators, nurse practitioners, or staff nurses. In most situations, books are appropriate for more than one audience, and all of these should be included in the review. Hill (1997) recommends that authors reviewing a book should take the perspective of different audiences and describe how the book could be used by each one. This avoids the tendency to review the book based on the author's own needs and background. For example, if the author is a nurse practitioner, a book may seem too basic for the reviewer's own practice, but if reviewed from the perspective of new graduates or staff nurses, it may be at the appropriate level.
- Assess if the content is up-to-date and reflects research findings if available.
- Review how the book is designed. Are there sufficient headings and subheadings? Are there visuals to support the content? For textbooks,

are strategies included to promote learning, such as chapter objectives and learning activities?

- Review the references. Are they current? If older references are included in the chapters, are they classic in the field? Does the book have references from other fields?
- Include the book price, its value, and if it is unique (Hill, 1997).

LETTER TO THE EDITOR

Whereas anyone can write a letter to the editor, not everyone can get it published. Journals and newspapers receive many letters, only some of which are published. Letters may be written to the journal's editor to provide an alternate perspective to an earlier article; they may sent to a newspaper to explain a topic to the public or present a viewpoint about an issue.

Not every journal publishes letters to the editor, so the author first should check the information for authors page or scan copies of the journal. If commenting on an article published earlier in the journal, the author should make this clear in the beginning of the letter. Huth (1999) recommended that words be carefully selected to avoid a personal attack on the authors of the article being critiqued. The writing style and format are similar to editorials. Because most journals limit the length of letters to the editor, the author should keep this in mind and prepare a letter that is short and to the point.

Authors also can send letters to newspapers and magazines. Carroll (1999) presented six tips for writing these letters: (1) be concise, (2) present only one topic, (3) clearly state the viewpoint, (4) state opinions directly, (5) if responding to comments made by others, do not use stereotypes for describing them, and (6) be accurate.

WRITING FOR CONSUMERS AND NONPROFESSIONAL AUDIENCES

Another type of writing is for consumers and nonprofessional audiences. Nurses have the background and education for writing health articles for the public, and they need to take the initiative to prepare these articles. Consumer magazines are a major source of health education for the public; these publications allow nurses to share their expertise with readers (Jimenez, 1991).

With this type of writing, the author needs to be clear about who reads the publication so that the content and writing can be geared to them. Examples can be used that are relevant to the readers. A manuscript on how to choose a primary care provider would have different examples if written for a magazine read by parents of young children compared with one geared to older readers. The other task is to avoid using technical terms and to develop the manuscript at a level that can be understood by readers without any health care background.

The author can begin by writing health pieces for newsletters and local newspapers. This provides experience in gearing the writing to a nonprofessional audience and deciding what information is most important to communicate to the public.

 ## WRITING CHAPTERS AND BOOKS

Preparing chapters and books represents a different form of writing because the author has more opportunity to provide background information and discuss related content, and with more pages allowed than in a manuscript for a journal. Whereas a journal manuscript may run 15 to 18 pages of text, a chapter may be 30 to 40 pages, depending on the book's length. Because of this, chapters allow for more discussion of the topic. They also provide an opportunity for the author to develop strategies to help readers learn the content, such as including learning activities with the chapter, bulleted lists emphasizing the key points, case scenarios showing how the content applies to clinical practice, and questions for discussion at the end of each chapter.

Whereas articles generally focus on one topic, books address multiple but related content areas. A book designed for use in an undergraduate course on nursing maternity patients contains the range of topics needed by students at this level to understand maternity nursing and gain the knowledge and skills for safe and competent practice. Even a book with a more specific focus, such as case management, will contain the content areas needed to understand and implement case management in varied clinical settings.

One consideration for faculty is that chapters and books are not refereed and often carry less weight in tenure and promotion decisions. Although the publisher will have experts review the prospectus, which is the plan for the book, and sometimes the finished product, this review generally is done to identify missing content, suggest changes in organization, or recommend different emphasis of chapters. These expert reviewers do not conduct a peer review, as is done with refereed publications. In some academic settings, tenure-track faculty are cautioned about focusing their writing on chapters and books rather than refereed articles.

Initial Contact With Publisher

The idea for a book may be initiated by the author, often the result of the author's inability to find a book for teaching a course or to meet a professional or personal need. In this situation, the author will approach different publishers to find one interested in publishing the work. Alternately, authors with known expertise may be asked by a publisher to write a book. In this instance, the publisher may not have a book in that content area to market to readers or faculty for courses. Usually, the acquisitions editor contacts the author to inquire about the author's interest.

Publishers include commercial firms that publish books in nursing, medicine, allied health, and other fields; organizations such as the American Nurses Association; and university presses. Some publishers have more experience with nursing books than others, and authors should have this information at hand when deciding on which publisher to contact about their ideas.

Types of Books

There are different types of books to consider. These include textbooks for students, which may be written for particular courses; resource books for nurses in practice, teaching, or administration; handbooks, which present abbreviated versions of content and are practical, such as handbooks on nursing diagnoses and interventions; manuals on procedures and technologies of care; case studies, usually in a specific clinical area such as critical care; and edited books containing chapters written by different authors and coordinated by an editor or editors. The problem with some edited books is the lack of consistency in the presentation of the content and writing style across chapters.

Another type of book is a monograph, which is a short book on a given topic such as group process. These generally are difficult to get published because of their specialized nature, and their commercial value may be minimal (Barnum, 1995).

Prospectus

Whether the author approaches the publisher with an idea or is contacted by the acquisitions editor or another representative of the publisher, the process begins with a literature search and completion of a prospectus. The prospectus is the proposal or plan for the book outlining its goals and how the author envisions the development of content.

Publishers have their own formats for preparing the prospectus, which generally include the following information:

- Purpose of the book and why it is needed
- List of chapters in the book and content of each
- Features of the book
- Contributors, if any, and which chapters they will prepare
- Intended readers, including the level of nursing students if it is a textbook

- Courses in which the book could be used and other market considerations
- Competition, including a review of every competing book on the market and statement as to why the proposed book would be better
- Timetable for its completion
- Size of the book, including total number of pages
- Sample chapter.

Authors should contact a publisher first, and if there is interest in the proposal, then prepare a prospectus for that publisher. It is risky to begin writing the manuscript without a publisher in case none can be found. It may be that the market is too small or there are too many books with the same content. Whereas the topic may be important to the author, the publisher may show minimal interest. In other cases, the publisher may be interested only if the focus changes considerably. Therefore, the author is advised to contact publishers before beginning to write.

Responsibilities of Author and Publisher

The prospectus then is sent to the publisher, who reviews it and, if interested, sends the author a contract. The contract is a legal document outlining the responsibilities of the author, or editor if a contributed book, and the publisher. The author is responsible for preparing the book and submitting it on time. The publisher is responsible for getting the book into production, copy editing the manuscript, designing the book, carrying out other details to produce it, and marketing it.

Some publishers send the completed book manuscript for external review to identify omissions of content and possible redundancies. Similar to journals, book authors receive edited versions of their manuscripts and page proofs to review.

Authors who serve as editors of contributed books have added responsibilities to define the content and length of each chapter for contributors, develop schedules for submission, and make sure that contributors adhere to them. With an edited book, format and writing style must be consistent across chapters. This may require rewriting by the editor.

Process of Writing Books

The process for writing a book is no different than other manuscripts, except for the length of the project and the need to stay on a strict time frame. When writing a book, the author must keep to deadlines and persevere or the book never will be completed. Techniques discussed in earlier chapters on preparing to write, organizing the writing project, and working with groups are important when writing a book. The author needs to view the writing project as a series of smaller "assignments," each with their own due dates for completion (Oermann, 1999). For large writing projects, deadlines must be met because lost time is difficult to make up. Display 7.2 provides tips for completing chapters, books, and similar writing projects that extend over a period of time.

SUMMARY

Clinical practice articles disseminate new knowledge and skills for patient care, provide information for nurses to stay current in clinical practice, and update them on new technologies and advances in care. With this type of article, nurses in one setting can describe their practice innovations for use and testing by nurses in other settings. They can discuss issues they faced in patient care and how they resolved those issues, and they can share nursing measures that worked and ones that did not work.

The process for writing a clinical article begins with an idea. From this idea, the author specifies the purpose of the manuscript and then identifies the intended readers. The intended reader of the article dictates the content included in it. In planning the content, the author takes into consideration the knowledge and background of the intended audience.

There is no standard format for writing clinical articles in contrast to research papers because it depends on the purpose of the manuscript. General

---

DISPLAY 7.2 **Tips for Completing Chapters and Books**

- Work on one chapter at a time.
- Develop an outline of topics to be covered in the chapter and organize them.
- Divide the topics into smaller, manageable parts.
- Treat each part as a separate writing project and assign a realistic due date to each part.
- Keep a running list of related activities that need to be completed for the chapter; assign due dates to these.
- Keep the due dates in a prominent place.
- Find your prime time for writing, when most creative, and guard it.
- Use other times of day for completing related writing activities, such as checking references.
- Learn to manage or avoid interruptions.
- Be persistent—complete each separate writing project that you identified on time.
- Repeat the process for each chapter.

Adapted from Oermann, M.H. (1999). Extensive writing projects: Tips for completing them on time. *Nurse Author & Editor, 9*(1), 8–10.

guidelines for writing clinical articles were presented in this chapter, including how to write the title, the abstract, the introduction and different types of lead-in paragraphs, and the body of the paper. Every clinical article ends with a conclusion that summarizes the information and its value to nurses in their own clinical practice.

Another type of manuscript relates to the professional role of the nurse. Rather than providing information applicable to patient care, the focus instead is on role development, performance, and evaluation.

What about issues in nursing? These papers analyze issues, why and how they developed, varied positions that can be taken, and multiple strategies for resolving them.

Other topics may be philosophical or may deal with theory development or testing. In writing philosophical and theoretical manuscripts, the author must be careful with how ideas are presented and ordered so that they are logical and sequenced appropriately. A sound argument must be presented to support ideas and defend them using theory and research.

The results of integrative reviews and meta-analyses also may be prepared for publication. For an integrative review article, the author identifies past research on a particular topic, critiques these studies, and then draws conclusions about the findings. Integrative review articles are important because they provide evidence for making decisions about clinical practice. A meta-analysis extends the critique of the research articles to include statistical analysis of the outcomes of similar studies.

Case reports provide new information on nursing practice and the care of patients with particular health problems through the presentation of an actual case. With some journals, nurses may be asked to write the editorial. Editorials may be issue oriented, summarize new developments in the field, or critically review an original paper in the journal. Nurses also might write book reviews describing what the book is about and addressing its quality, letters to the editor, and articles for consumers and nonprofessional audiences.

The last section of the chapter addresses writing books in nursing. Whether the author approaches the publisher with an idea or is contacted by the publisher to write a book, the process begins with a literature search and completion of a prospectus. The prospectus is the proposal for the book outlining its goals and how the author envisions the development of content. Typical content in the prospectus is discussed in the chapter.

Many of the situations in which nurses find themselves lend to writing for publication. Nurses need to take advantage of these opportunities so their ideas are communicated to and used by others.

REFERENCES

Advances in Nursing Science. (2000). Author's guide. [On-line]. Available: *http://www. nursing.uconn.edu/plchinn/ANSathgd.html*. Accessed November 8, 2000.

American Medical Association. (1998). *Manual of style: A guide for authors and editors* (9th ed.). Baltimore: Williams & Wilkins.

American Psychological Association (APA). (1994). *Publication manual of the American Psychological Association* (4th ed.). Washington, DC: APA.

Ashworth, P. (1998). Nurses now read more: What about writing too? *Intensive and Critical Care Nursing, 14,* 107.

Barnum, B.S. (1995). *Writing and getting published.* New York: Springer.

Beck, C.T. (1999). Facilitating the work of a meta-analyst. *Research in Nursing & Health, 22,* 523–530.

Bell, F.J. (1998). Reviewing the literature: A student's perspective. *Journal of Child Health Care, 2*(3), 122–127

Beyea, S.C., & Nicoll, L.H. (1998). Writing an integrative review. *AORN Journal, 67,* 877–880.

Black, J. (1996). Writing for publication: Advice to potential authors. *Plastic Surgical Nursing, 16,* 90–93.

Carroll, P. (1999). Getting heard: Writing opinion pieces for the newspaper. *Nurse Author & Editor, 9*(3), 4, 7–8.

Carson, P.P. (2000). Adrenal crisis. *American Journal of Nursing, 100*(7), 49–50.

Clinical Nurse Specialist. (2000). Description. [On-line]. Available: *http://www. nursingcenter.com/journals/index.cfm.* Accessed November 7, 2000.

Fondiller, S. (1994). Writing for publication. *American Journal of Nursing, 94*(8), 62–65.

Harrison, L.L. (1999). Pulling it together: The importance of integrative research reviews and meta-analyses in nursing. *Journal of Advanced Nursing, 24,* 224–225.

Henderson-Martin, B. (2000). No more surprises: Screening patients for alcohol abuse. *American Journal of Nursing, 100*(9), 26–32.

Hill, K. (1997). Book reviewing: Keeping the audience in mind. *Nurse Author & Editor, 7*(1), 4, 7–8.

Huth, E.J. (1999). *Writing and publishing in medicine* (3rd ed.). Baltimore: Lippincott Williams & Wilkins.

International Committee of Medical Journal Editors. (1997). Uniform requirements for manuscripts submitted to biomedical journals. *Annals of Internal Medicine, 126,* 36–47. Also available at http://www.icmje.org/.

Jimenez, S.L. (1991). Consumer journalism: A unique nursing opportunity. *Image: Journal of Nursing Scholarship, 23,* 47–49.

Johnson, S.H. (1997). The five "do's" to writing a book review: The editor's view. *Nurse Author & Editor, 7*(1), 7.

Jones, S. (2000). Neonatal wound dehiscence and the subsequent healing process: A case study. *Ostomy/Wound Management, 46*(6), 42–45, 48–50.

Journal of Nursing Administration. (2000). Description. [On-line]. Available: *http://www.nursingcenter.com/journals/index.cfm.* Accessed November 7, 2000.

Journal of Obstetric, Gynecologic, and Neonatal Nursing. (2000). Author guidelines. [On-line]. Available: *http://www.nursingcenter.com/journals/index.cfm.* Accessed November 10, 2000.

McHale, J.E., & Barth, M.M. (2000). Nursing care after pneumonectomy in patients with invasive pulmonary aspergillosis. *Critical Care Nurse, 20*(1), 37–44.

Nursing Science Quarterly. (2000). About the journal. [On-line]. Available: *http://www.sagepub.co.uk/frame.html?http://www.sagepub.co.uk/journals/details/j0289. html*. Accessed November 7, 2000.

Oermann, M.H. (1999). Extensive writing projects: Tips for completing them on time. *Nurse Author & Editor, 9*(1), 8–10.

Online Journal of Issues in Nursing. (2000). Journal focus. [On-line]. Available: *http://www.nursingworld.org/ojin/admin/ojinwrtr.htm#JF*. Accessed November 7, 2000.

Rosswurm, M.A., & Larrabee, J.H. (1999). A model for change to evidence-based practice. *Image: Journal of Nursing Scholarship, 31*, 317–322.

Sanford, R.C. (2000). Caring through relation and dialogue: A nursing perspective for patient education. *Advances in Nursing Science, 22*(3), 1–15.

Stepanski, L.M. (1999). The nurse as rhetorician. *Journal of Intravenous Nursing, 22*, 94–99.

The Nurse Practitioner. (2000). Information for authors. [On-line]. Available: *http://www.tnpj.com/np/journal/authors.html*. Accessed November 7, 2000.

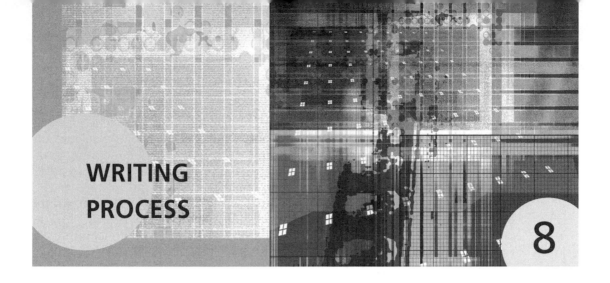

WRITING
PROCESS

8

At this point in the process of writing, the author has identified the type of manuscript, the purpose of the paper, potential journals, and the audience to which the paper will be geared. The author has obtained author guidelines, has conducted or updated the literature review, has completed other preparations for writing, and now is ready to begin writing the manuscript.

Writing for publication requires careful planning, organization, and personal strategies to keep on target until the paper is completed. It cannot be done haphazardly. With an outline—even if brief—and materials assembled, the author can move quickly into writing the first draft. The author should plan on revising the draft several times until satisfied with the final copy. This chapter focuses on organizing the content, including how to develop an outline, and writing the first draft of the manuscript.

PREPARATIONS FOR WRITING

Before beginning the outline, the author completes other preparations to facilitate the writing process and eliminate unnecessary distractions. These preparations include reviewing the author guidelines for the journal to clarify the format and other requirements; gathering materials about the project, innovation, or practices described in the manuscript; and assembling analyses of data and other information about the research project. These preliminary activities are important to allow authors to focus on their writing once they begin rather than on time-consuming, and sometimes distracting, tasks such as finding evidence needed to support ideas, locating statistical analyses of data, and checking references. The goal is to assemble all materials before writing the first draft.

The literature review should be available if references need to be checked during the writing phase. No writer, even an experienced one, can rely on memory to cite a reference in a manuscript. Authors even in high-quality journals make too many errors in their reference lists. This can be avoided by carefully checking each reference when preparing the manuscript.

This is not the time to learn how to use a new word-processing program, develop tables, or type references. When the author begins to write, all of these activities should have been completed, enabling the author to concentrate on preparing the first draft.

Review Purpose and Audience

Before writing the first draft, the author should spend time planning how to approach the topic. Reviewing the purpose of the manuscript is the first step in this planning. It often is helpful to record the purpose on a note card placed in a visible spot as a way of keeping the manuscript focused on this main point. The author should be able to track the main point from the beginning of the manuscript to the end.

The author then should think about the intended readers. What is their level of knowledge and expertise? Why is the article important to them? Knowing the intended readers, combined with recognizing the purpose of the manuscript, guides the author in writing the first draft. If the primary audience is nurses in the same specialty field or a related one, authors are essentially writing for their peers and therefore are able to use technical and highly specialized language in the writing. Examples from nursing practice and case studies that focus on nursing care would be easily understood by readers and therefore appropriate for inclusion in the manuscript.

The primary audience of other journals, though, may be readers from different disciplines. The *Joint Commission Journal on Quality Improvement* is a journal that provides information on measuring, assessing, and improving the performance of health care organizations. When writing for this journal, authors would avoid using terms and examples unique to nursing and instead would write so that any professional involved in measuring and improving performance could understand.

Review Writing Style of Journal

In writing the manuscript, the author needs to use a writing style consistent with the journal. Otherwise, the manuscript may be rejected or the author will need to rewrite the paper to fit the journal's style.

Formal Writing Style

Writing style can be categorized in different ways. One way is to classify styles of writing as formal or informal. A formal style is more scientific and scholarly. An example of a formal writing style follows:

> Despite extensive research on defining and measuring health care quality, less attention has been given to consumers' views of quality health care. Most studies examine the type of information needed by consumers to choose between varied health plans, but whether consumers understand this information and if they will use it in making health care decisions have not been established through research.

Formal writing style often uses the passive voice, where the action happens to the subject instead of the subject initiating the action. The following example demonstrates passive voice:

> A new teaching plan was developed to standardize teaching in the clinic and improve educational outcomes of patients.

Informal Writing Style

An informal writing style uses more active-voice sentences, which state who or what the subject is doing. Many readers find sentences written in active voice easier to read and understand. Active-voice writing also keeps readers' interest (Pearsall, 1997). The earlier sentence written with passive voice can be rewritten with active voice by adding the subject, that is, the persons who developed the new teaching plan:

> *The nurses in the clinic* developed a new teaching plan to standardize teaching and improve educational outcomes of patients.

With an informal style, personal pronouns sometimes are used such as "I" and "we." Using personal pronouns in writing often goes hand in hand with active-voice sentences. For instance, the example sentence just given might begin with a personal pronoun:

> *We* developed a new teaching plan to standardize teaching in the clinic and improve educational outcomes of patients.

Similarly, informal writing style often uses the personal pronoun "you" to engage the reader in the topic and personalize the information. In the following example of an informal writing style, the personal pronoun "you" is used:

> *You* can help the patient to break down his overall stress into separate concerns that can be addressed one at a time. *You* can also refer the patient to the nurse practitioner if needed.

OUTLINE

An outline is a general plan of the content to be included in the manuscript and its organization (Oermann, 1999b; 2000). Outlines may be formal, such as one developed using Roman numerals, or informal, such as a list of topics in order. Regardless of whether the outline is formal or informal, it enables the author to specify content areas to include in the manuscript and decide how to logically organize these topics so that information is clear to readers. Outlining is essential to provide a logical structure to the manuscript and guide the author in writing the first draft (Muscari, 1998).

Some authors prefer not to develop an outline, but even experienced authors may drift in their writing and find as they near the end of a manuscript that certain content areas were omitted or that the organization was unclear. It is easier and quicker to revise an outline than a draft of an entire paper, so the time devoted to outlining is worth it in the long run.

The author should view the outline as a working document; the outline is not a final product but instead is a tool to aid writing the first draft. Some authors find it helpful before writing the draft to review the outline a few days after its initial development to assess if changes are needed and to add details to the content.

Advantages of Outlines

Oermann (2000) identified five advantages of outlining before starting to write the first draft. An outline:

- Provides a way of planning content to include in the manuscript and deciding how to organize it
- Suggests headings and subheadings that might be used with the manuscript
- Allows the author to focus on the content when writing the draft rather than how to organize it
- Keeps the author on target
- Assists the author in developing an argument to support a position in the manuscript.

Types of Outlines

Outlines may be formal or informal. A formal outline uses a standard format such as Roman numerals or decimals. Authors can prepare an outline themselves with Roman numerals or decimals or can use the outline mode in the word-processing program. For instance, Microsoft Word's outline view automatically formats the outline and assigns numbers. When changes are made in the level of the outline, the content automatically is renumbered. For some authors, though, it is easier to develop an outline themselves rather than use word-processing software.

When outlining using the computer, Johnson (2000) suggests opening two document windows at a time: one for the outline, and one for the manuscript text. The author then can follow the outline while writing the manuscript; topics from the outline often make good headings and subheadings for the manuscript and can be copied easily to the manuscript text.

An informal outline is a list of topics and subtopics to be included in the manuscript in the order to be discussed. Often, the author uses indentation to represent more specific levels of content. For many authors, an informal outline of headings and subheadings and how they will be organized is sufficient (Pearsall, 1997).

The amount of detail to include in the outline depends on the author and what style best facilitates writing the manuscript. There is not one correct way to develop an outline. All authors should develop a style of outlining that best meets their own needs. For some authors, developing a detailed and formal outline is essential to stay on target and to avoid having to think about how to structure the content while writing. For these persons, outlining saves valuable time later, when writing the first draft. For others, a brief list of topics to be covered in order in the manuscript is sufficient to guide writing. Regardless of the format, it is valuable to use the same type of outlining for each writing project (Houp, Pearsall, & Tebeaux, 1998).

Examples of outlines are found in Displays 8.1 and 8.2. Display 8.1 shows an outline and subsequent text developed from that outline. Display 8.2 is a sample outline for a research manuscript.

Techniques for Outlining

Before beginning the outline, the author should review quickly the materials gathered, making notes on how the material might be grouped into topics and how the topics might be arranged (Oermann, 1999a). This gives the author a general sense of the organization of the content.

If unsure how to organize the content, one technique is to record key content areas on separate index cards. This can be done while the author is reviewing the materials in preparation for beginning the manuscript. Each index card should have a major content area listed on it; these content areas represent the main topics to be covered in the manuscript. The author then can arrange the cards in a logical order, rearranging as needed until comfortable with the organization. Subtopics can be recorded with the relevant content area and then organized logically. This technique allows the author to eas-

OUTLINE FOR ARTICLE: "DEVELOPING A TEACHING PORTFOLIO"

I. Uses of teaching portfolios
   A. Documenting teaching effectiveness in nursing education programs
   B. Promotion
   C. Tenure
   D. Reappointment
   E. Merit
II. Quality of teaching, research, service, and clinical practice
   A. Depends on mission and purposes of nursing program
   B. Emphasis on teaching by program
III. Definition of teaching portfolio
   A. Compilation of carefully selected materials that describe faculty's teaching activities
      1. Classroom
      2. Clinical practice
      3. Learning laboratory
   B. Materials chosen by teacher
   C. Demonstrates full range of teaching competencies

ARTICLE: "DEVELOPING A TEACHING PORTFOLIO"

Teaching portfolios are being used more widely for documenting teaching effectiveness in nursing education programs. Promotion, tenure, reappointment, and merit decisions are based on an assessment of the quality of teaching, research, service, and clinical practice depending on the mission and purposes of the nursing program. Documenting the quality of teaching in the classroom, in clinical practice, and in the learning laboratory through student evaluations of teaching alone negates other sources of information about the teacher and the context within which the teaching has occurred. Teaching portfolios provide a solution to this issue because they allow faculty to compile materials that more fully represent the scope and quality of their instruction and supervision of students.

What is a Teaching Portfolio?

A teaching portfolio is a compilation of carefully selected materials that describe the faculty's teaching activities in the classroom, clinical practice, and other settings. Melland and Volden (1996) described portfolios in nursing as an approach to documenting teaching effectiveness based on materials chosen, presented, and organized by the teacher. The goal of the teaching portfolio is to describe through this documentation the full range of teaching competencies of the faculty over a period of time (Murray, 1994; Urbach, 1992). The materials selected by the teacher suggest the scope and quality of teaching beyond student ratings of teaching effectiveness.

From Oermann, M.H. (1999). Developing a teaching portfolio. *Journal of Professional Nursing, 15,* 224. Reprinted by permission of W.B. Saunders.

DISPLAY 8.2	Outline for Research Manuscript

Introduction
  Extensive research on defining and measuring quality of health care
  Limited attention to consumers' perspectives of quality care
  Purposes
    Identify importance to consumers of indicators of quality health care and nursing care
    Examine relationships of health status and demographic variables to consumers' views
Methods
  Exploratory design
  239 consumers, convenience sample
  How selected (waiting rooms of clinics and neighborhoods)
  Instruments
    Quality Health Care Questionnaire
    SF-36
Results
  Indicators of quality health care most important to consumers (Table 1)
  Indicators of quality nursing care most important to consumers (See Table 1)
  Differences based on race, income, and educational level (Table 2)
  Correlations of indicator ratings and health status (SF-36) (Table 3)
Discussion
  Consistency of findings with other studies
  Important implications for teaching patients in clinics

ily change the outline until it represents the best order in the author's judgment.

To arrive at a general organization, the author can record ideas about the content of the paper in the form of a map (Zilm, 1998). A concept map is a graphic or pictorial arrangement of key concepts and their interrelationships (Gaberson & Oermann, 1999). Mapping concepts visually helps authors to connect key ideas and organize them logically. The main idea is put in the middle of the map, with other ideas grouped around it. After the ideas are written down, the author can add numbers and letters to show their logical order and can use this as a guide to organize the content (Matthews, Bowen, & Matthews, 1996). Figure 8-1 provides an example of a beginning map for the article on developing a teaching portfolio outlined in Display 8.1.

Main Topic in Beginning of Outline

In the beginning of the outline, the author should state the main topic or content area. Stating the main idea early helps keep the writing focused on the

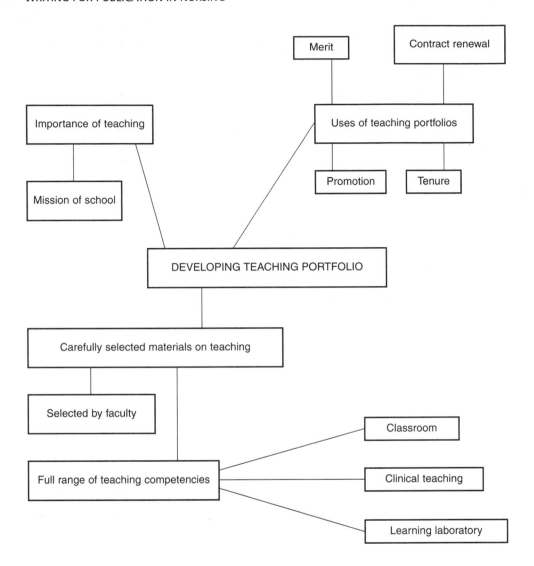

Figure 8-1. Map of ideas for manuscript.

purpose of the manuscript (Oermann, 2000). This also is important when writing the first draft because the main point should be highlighted in the introduction to the paper.

Outline as Time Management Tool

An outline has the advantages described earlier but also serves as a time management tool. With the outline, the author can separate writing the manuscript into smaller, more manageable steps and can assign a due date to each section. This helps the author to monitor progress in completing the paper and also provides reinforcement when a small section is completed.

When time for writing is limited, it often is helpful to plan on completing small sections of content at a time, using the dates on the outline as a way of monitoring progress. Most authors need clear due dates to finish their writing project, and these should be realistic, considering time and other constraints.

 ## FIRST DRAFT

Each author develops a way of writing—what works best for them. With a well thought-out outline and materials available that might be needed during the writing, the author is ready to begin the draft. The draft rarely is written all at once. Instead, the author should find the best time for writing and work on the draft over the next few weeks. The author should be careful not to extend the time for writing the draft for too long. When this happens, it is difficult to keep track of ideas and remain motivated about the writing project.

In preparing the first draft, the author should write fast to get the ideas on paper. This is not the time to be concerned about grammar, spelling, punctuation, and writing style. These will be revised later. Worrying about these while writing the first draft may interfere with thinking about how to present the content (Oermann, 1999b; Zilm, 1998). The goal with the first draft is to get the ideas on paper, using the outline for organizing them.

With the outline, the author should be able to start at the beginning of the manuscript with the main idea and write through each section to the end. Content can be reordered if needed by modifying the outline. Some authors, though, do not write each section of the manuscript in order. With experience, authors develop their own styles of writing and techniques for completing writing projects.

Fondiller (1999) suggested that beginning authors take too long to get started and write too slowly and tediously, pausing frequently to reread and edit what was written (p. 81). Instead, the author should write fast to get the content "on paper" and reread and edit later.

Title and Abstract

Some authors write the title and abstract first (Huth, 1999), whereas others wait until the first draft is completed. Because the title conveys the purpose of the paper and the abstract includes the main ideas in each section of it, writing these first may help the author to clarify the main points to be conveyed in the paper. Both the title and abstract may need to be revised later, so the author should consider these as a first draft. For others, it is easier to record the purpose of the paper on something tangible, such as an index card, and write the title and abstract after the first draft is completed.

Sheridan and Dowdney (1997) suggested writing a working title in the form of a statement first, then revising it into a question. The rest of the content then answers this question.

Reference Citations in Draft

In the citation-sequence system, references in the reference list are numbered according to the order in which they first appear in the text. Rather than citing the author's name and date of publication in the text, a reference number is used instead. For instance, this system of referencing appears in the following example:

> Teaching portfolios are being used more widely for documenting teaching effectiveness in nursing education programs.[1]

In the reference list at the end of the paper, number 1 refers to this particular reference by Oermann in 1999. Only the number, though, is listed in the text of the paper.

In the name-year system, which is the reference format used by the American Psychological Association (1994), the author's name and date of publication are cited in the body instead of a number. References then are organized alphabetically on the reference list. For example,

> Teaching portfolios are being used more widely for documenting teaching effectiveness in nursing education programs (Oermann, 1999).

Even if the journal selected uses the citation-sequence system, the author's last name and date of the publication should be recorded in the drafts of the manuscript. The references can be numbered later. If numbers are assigned before the final copy, they need to be changed every time content is shifted and a reference is added or deleted. To make it easier to correct the reference format with the final manuscript, the author can insert a symbol before each citation in the text and can use the "find" function in the word processing program. With this function, the author can move quickly through the document to find the references and then replace them with a number.

If using a bibliographic management program, references are marked in the text and then converted to the proper reference format later. The author should learn how to use this software before writing the first draft.

Even though this is the first draft, authors should be careful about how they cite references to avoid errors. Sometimes, in an effort to quickly write the first draft and get ideas expressed, authors make notations about references as a way of remembering to include them in the manuscript but later forget to check them for accuracy.

Preparing the Draft

Authors need to find their own techniques for preparing the draft. Some authors write best on paper first, then type it or have someone else type it; others prefer to compose the draft directly on the computer. Regardless of the process used, each draft should be numbered and dated. This allows the author to refer back to earlier drafts. If preparing the manuscript on a word processor, one easy way to number and date the drafts is by inserting this information in a header or footer. This is shown in Display 8.3.

If writing alone and working from the beginning section to the end, pages can be numbered sequentially. However, some authors write sections "out of order," and in these instances, a system should be devised for numbering pages within each section. Otherwise, the author may be faced with a situation in which pages were printed from the computer for review without a clear indication as to their order. If co-authors are submitting drafts of sections to the primary author, a system should be devised for noting the name of the contributor, numbering and dating the draft, and numbering the pages of the contributed section.

Line Numbering and Displaying Revisions of Draft

DISPLAY 8.3 **Labeling Drafts**

[Teaching Portfolio, 1st draft, 7/12/01]

Documenting the quality of teaching in the classroom, in clinical practice, and in the learning laboratory through student evaluations of teaching alone negates other sources of information about the teacher and the context within which the teaching has occurred. Teaching portfolios provide a solution to this issue because they allow faculty to compile materials that more fully represent the scope and quality of their instruction and supervision of students. More and more nursing programs are using teaching portfolios for documenting teaching effectiveness.

[Teaching Portfolio, 2nd draft, 8/27/01]

Teaching portfolios are being used more widely for documenting teaching effectiveness in nursing education programs. Promotion, tenure, reappointment, and merit decisions are based on an assessment of the quality of teaching, research, service, and clinical practice depending on the mission and purposes of the nursing program. Teaching portfolios allow faculty to compile materials that more fully represent the scope and quality of their instruction and supervision of students.

When writing in a group and exchanging sections of the manuscript for critique, it is helpful to number the lines. The lines can be numbered automatically by the wordprocessing program, enabling co-authors to communicate more easily where changes are needed. For example,

254   An important document in the teaching portfolio is the faculty's
255   philosophy of teaching. The beliefs and assumptions in your
256   philosophy guide the design of the course and clinical practicum,
257   selection of teaching methods and assignments, structure of the
258   clinical experience, evaluation strategies, and grading practices.
259   The philosophy, therefore, sets the framework for the . . .

With line numbering an author can indicate that "your" in line 255 should be replaced with "the teacher's."

Other word processing functions for showing draft revisions include using annotations, inserting comments, and marking the revisions with different colors while editing. Manuscripts then can be sent electronically to co-authors, indicating the queries and suggesting revisions in the draft using one of these techniques.

Number of Drafts

There is no set number of drafts to write until the finished product becomes satisfactory. Some authors need to revise their drafts more than others. In the first few drafts, authors should continue to focus on expressing the content clearly and thoroughly. Only when satisfied with the content should the author begin to revise grammar, punctuation, spelling, and writing style. The key in writing the first and early drafts is to get the content on paper and organize it effectively. Keegan (1999) suggested printing the first draft, then reading it again in a few days to determine if content has been omitted.

The first draft should include all of the essential content, even if it is repetitious in some sections. As Fondiller (1999) pointed out, it is easier to delete unwanted content later than to fill in areas done too briefly.

There comes a time, however, when the author needs to stop modifying the content, or the drafting phase never will end. The author should avoid trying to write a finished manuscript as a first draft and instead should focus on including the essential content.

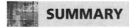 **SUMMARY**

Before beginning the first draft, the author completes preparations to facilitate the writing process and eliminate unnecessary distractions. These preparations include reviewing the author guidelines for the journal to clarify the

format and other requirements; gathering materials about the project, innovation, or practices described in the manuscript; and assembling analyses of data and other information about the research project. The goal is to assemble all materials before writing the first draft.

After reviewing the purpose of the manuscript and intended audience, the author writes an outline, which is a general plan of the content to be included in the manuscript and its organization. Outlines may be formal, such as one developed using Roman numerals, or informal, such as topics listed in order.

Using the outline, the author writes the first draft. The important principle here is to get the ideas on paper. This is not the time to be concerned about grammar, spelling, punctuation, and writing style—these are revised later. The goal with the first draft is to present the content following the format of the outline.

There is no set number of drafts to write until satisfied with the finished product. Some authors need to revise their drafts more than others. In the first few drafts, authors should continue to focus on expressing the content clearly and thoroughly. When satisfied with the content, the author revises the grammar, punctuation, spelling, and writing style, as discussed in Chapter 9.

REFERENCES

American Psychological Association (APA). (1994). *Publication manual of the American Psychological Association* (4th ed.). Washington, DC: APA.

Fondiller, S.H. (1999). *The writer's workbook* (2nd ed.). Sudbury, MA: Jones & Bartlett.

Gaberson, K., & Oermann, M.H. (1999). Clinical teaching strategies in nursing education. New York: Springer.

Houp, K.W., Pearsall, T.E., & Tebeaux, E. (1998). *Reporting technical information* (9th ed.). Boston: Allyn & Bacon.

Huth, E.J. (1999). *Writing and publishing in medicine* (3rd ed.). Baltimore: Lippincott Williams & Wilkins.

Johnson, S.H. (2000). Refining outlining skills: Part II. The computer methods. *Nurse Author & Editor, 10*(3), 1–3.

Keegan, L. (1999). Assessing your publication potential. *Seminars in Perioperative Nursing, 8*(1), 3–6.

Matthews, J.R., Bowen, J.M., & Matthews, R.W. (1996). *Successful scientific writing: A step-by-step guide for biomedical scientists*. Cambridge: Cambridge University Press.

Muscari, M.E. (1998). Do the write thing: Writing the clinically focused article. *Journal of Pediatric Health Care, 12*, 236–241.

Oermann, M.H. (1999a). Extensive writing projects: Tips for completing them on time. *Nurse Author & Editor, 9*(1), 8–10.

Oermann, M.H. (1999b). Writing for publication as an advanced practice nurse. *Nursing Connections, 12*(3), 5–13.

Oermann, M.H. (2000). Refining outlining skills: Part I. The topic or sentence method. *Nurse Author & Editor, 10*(2), 4, 7–8.

Pearsall, T.E. (1997). *The elements of technical writing.* Boston: Allyn and Bacon.

Sheridan, D.R., & Dowdney, D.L. (1997). *How to write and publish articles in nursing* (2nd ed.). New York: Springer.

Zilm, G. (1998). The SMART way: An introduction to writing for nurses. Toronto: Harcourt Brace & Company.

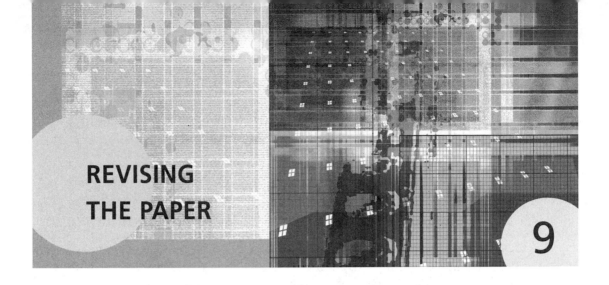

REVISING
THE PAPER

9

In Chapter 8, guidelines were provided for preparing to write the manuscript, planning the content, developing an outline, and writing the first draft. In writing the first draft, the author focuses on presenting and organizing the content rather than on grammar, punctuation, spelling, and writing style.

This chapter describes the steps in revising the content and organization of the paper and then revising the writing structure and style. Some principles are provided for improving how the paper is written, but the chapter does not address all aspects of prose structure and style that are important in writing for publication.

REVISING THE FIRST DRAFT

The goal in writing the first draft of the manuscript is to present the essential content in a logical order. With this goal in mind, the initial revisions of the draft should focus on modifying the content and how it is organized, not on grammar, punctuation, spelling, and writing style (Oermann, 1999a, 1999b). Once the content is revised sufficiently and approved by co-authors, then the draft is reviewed for writing structure and style.

There is no set number of drafts to write until satisfied with the content and its organization. Some authors need to revise their drafts more than others. At least three drafts are likely to be needed to ensure that the content is accurate, is organized clearly, and is covered adequately in the paper and that nonessential content has been eliminated.

Because the author invests much time in writing the first draft and may be unsure where revisions are needed, it may be beneficial for some authors to wait before revising the content and organization. The author might print the first draft, then read it again in a few days or a week to determine if content has been omitted and to decide if it needs to be reorganized. During that time, the author may lose some attachment to the writing and be more objective when rereading it (Black, 1995).

Goals of Revision: Content and Organization

In revising the content and its organization, authors become their own peer reviewers and editors. Authors need to be critical of their own work. They should view the draft as a "work in progress," which needs to be revised, rather than as a finished product. Otherwise, authors may be unwilling to make changes that are essential to improving the manuscript.

The principles described earlier for preparing each section of the manuscript may be used as a framework for revising the first and later drafts in terms of content and organization. Display 9.1 provides a list of questions for authors to use in revising the paper.

Review the Title

If the author developed a working title, this can be reviewed first. The title should capture the purpose of the manuscript and for research manuscripts should indicate the objective of the study. Some authors write the draft first, then develop the title; others write the title first with the understanding that it may be revised as the paper is developed. Regardless of when the title is prepared, at some point during the revision of the draft, the author should critique the title to determine if it needs to be revised.

Review the Abstract

Similar to the title, authors write the abstract at different points in time. Some prepare a draft of the abstract before writing the manuscript, whereas others wait until the first draft is completed. In reviewing the abstract, the author examines if it adequately summarizes the purpose of the paper and indicates the most important content within the length allowed by the journal. For research manuscripts, the abstract should describe the study purpose and background, methods, and findings.

Review the Text

In reviewing the main body of the paper, the author begins by reading the introductory section. For research manuscripts, the introduction should indicate what was known about the topic, what questions remained, and how the current project answered those questions. For manuscripts on clinical practice, a good introduction conveys why the paper is important to the nurse's

| DISPLAY 9.1 | **Revising Content and Organization: Questions to Ask** |

TITLE

Does the title communicate the purpose of the manuscript?
Is the title informative?
Is it accurate?
Is the title too long? If so, what words can be deleted?

ABSTRACT

Does the abstract summarize the most important content in the paper?
Does the abstract of a research manuscript describe the background, purpose, methods, and findings of the study within the length allowed?

TEXT

Is the purpose of the paper clear and introduced early in the discussion?
Does the introduction explain why the content is important and how it will improve readers' knowledge or skill?
Can the main purpose be traced from the introduction to the end of the text?
Is important literature reviewed and synthesized?
Is the literature review relevant for the goals of the paper and journal?
Is the literature current?
Is any content missing?
Is there any content that is repetitive in the text?
What content can be omitted from the paper?
Is the content accurate?
Is the content sequenced clearly and logically?
Is it clear how the content may be used in the nurse's own work and setting?

REFERENCES

Are all references essential?
Have any important references been omitted?
Are the references consistent with the citations in the paper?

TABLES AND FIGURES

Do tables and figures display specific data that supplement and support the text?
Are they consistent with the text?
Is each table and figure essential?

HEADINGS AND SUBHEADINGS

Are the headings and subheadings effective in organizing the content of the manuscript?
Are they substantive, informing readers of the content that follows?
Do they provide transition from one topic to the next?
Are the correct levels of headings and subheadings used to reflect the importance of the content area?

(continued)

DISPLAY 9.1	Revising Content and Organization: Questions to Ask *(Continued)*

ADDITIONAL QUESTIONS FOR RESEARCH MANUSCRIPTS

Are the purposes of the study, research questions, and hypotheses stated clearly for readers?

Are the gaps in knowledge and limitations of prior studies emphasized to provide support for the current study?

Does the methods section adequately describe the study design, subjects, measures, procedures, and data analysis?

Does the results section present the findings of the study, addressing the original purposes of the research?

Are the main findings presented first?

Are the findings presented without discussion, which is provided in the subsequent section of the paper?

Are the results described accurately and precisely?

Are statistics reported correctly, using conventional format?

Does the discussion section interpret the results and explain what the findings mean in terms of the purpose of the study?

Are inconsistencies with prior research addressed?

Are implications of the study discussed?

own practice. The reader should know the purpose of the paper from reading the introductory section of the text. McConnell (1999) suggested getting readers' interest through anecdotes that illustrate the theme of the paper, a dramatic pronouncement, a compelling statistic, or a strong problem statement.

After critiquing the introduction, the author then is ready to review the rest of the text. First, the author should reread the draft to determine if content is missing. A section of content may have been missed in the outline, or in writing the paper, the author may have failed to elaborate sufficiently about a particular topic. To assess if content needs to be added, the author should read the draft as a whole without interruptions. Otherwise, the sequence of content and possible gaps in it may not be apparent.

Second, the text should be reviewed to eliminate repetitive content and to assess if any content can be omitted considering the purpose of the paper. In writing the first draft, authors often repeat ideas in different sections of the manuscript and frequently include more content than is essential. Any content that does not contribute substantially to the paper should be deleted (Muscari, 1998). The author is better off having prepared a shorter, precisely written manuscript than a longer one with content that is not essential to the goals of the paper. Entire sections or paragraphs of the manuscript may need to be eliminated; if so, the author should save the deleted content in a separate file in case it is needed later.

Because the author has devoted much time and effort to writing the first draft, it sometimes is difficult to delete content. The author, however, should be willing to make these changes to improve the manuscript.

Third, once the author has revised the content of the draft, the next step is to assess its organization or structure. Although an outline was used for writing the draft, the content in the outline may not have been structured clearly, or the author may have strayed from the outline in writing the draft. The author also may find that the broad organization of content is consistent with the outline and is clear, but the content within each section of the paper needs reorganization. For research papers using the IMRAD (Introduction, Methods, Results, and Discussion) format, the broad content areas are predetermined, but how the content is organized within each of these sections should be evaluated.

Fourth, the accuracy of the paper should be reviewed. For research papers, the author should check the accuracy of the data reported in the manuscript, statistical results, and conclusions reached from the findings. Each statement in the draft should be reread for accuracy and to decide whether it is supported adequately by the discussion.

Fifth, the end of the manuscript should bring the ideas to a close, summarizing the main points covered in the paper. The author should check that the manuscript does not end in midair when the last point planned for the discussion was addressed (McConnell, 1999). New concepts should not be introduced at the end, and the author should be able to trace the development of the main points of the paper from the beginning through the end. A few sentences usually are sufficient to summarize the conclusions from the paper and highlight the implications of the content for practice, teaching, administration, and future research.

Review References

The author should remember that the literature review in a paper provides the background information for readers but is not intended to be an exhaustive review of every article on a topic. In reviewing the references, the author should ask whether they are essential to support the goals of the paper and are consistent with the intended journal and readers. Unnecessary references should be omitted. When citing support for a statement, key references should be used rather than a long list of citations.

Review Tables and Figures

Consistent with eliminating unnecessary content, the author should review each table and figure to determine if it is essential to the paper. Some tables may be omitted because they duplicate the content in the text, or they may be developed as a result of revisions in the content. Tables and figures should supplement the text, not duplicate it. This is a good time for the author to recheck numerical data in the table for accuracy and consistency with the information reported in the text.

Headings and Subheadings

Headings and subheadings emphasize for readers the content covered in each section of the manuscript. They give structure to the paper, provide transition from one topic to the next, inform readers of the content that follows, and suggest the importance of each subject area. Headings of the same level typically represent topics of equal importance (American Psychological Association [APA], 1994). The revision of the paper provides an opportunity for the author to add headings and subheadings to the manuscript, if not done already, or to review those written.

Headings and subheadings often are identified by using the outline developed for the manuscript. For research papers following the IMRAD format, the headings are predetermined, although the author may choose to insert subheadings within these general areas. For nonresearch papers, though, the headings and subheadings are important to organize the content and indicate for readers the topics that follow. Day (1998) views headings as signposts to direct the readers through the paper. By dividing the manuscript into sections, headings also make the paper more attractive visually.

Headings and subheadings can be short sentences, phrases, single words, or questions. The key to writing them is to identify accurately the content contained in that section (Pearsall, 1997). Displays 9.2 and 9.3 present two documents, the first without headings and the second with them. Display 9.3 shows how headings improve readability and make the organization clearer for readers.

Journals use varied levels of headings; the author should review sample articles in the journal to determine the levels typically included in its publications. Often, two levels of headings are sufficient to provide organization to the manuscript. When additional levels are indicated, the author can consult the style manual for placement and typing.

Guidelines for preparing the headings and subheadings are as follows:

1. Develop substantive headings that inform readers of the content in the section that follows.
2. Write headings and subheadings as short sentences, phrases, single words, or questions.
3. Do not use a heading for the introduction because the first part of the manuscript is assumed to be the introductory section.
4. Avoid having only one subsection in a section, similar to principles for outlining (American Medical Association [AMA], 1998; APA, 1994).

DISPLAY 9.2 **Sample Document Without Headings**

An important area of current research focuses on providing quality information to consumers. Despite extensive research on defining and measuring the quality of health care, less attention has been given to consumers' perspectives of quality care. Most of the studies examine the type of information valuable in choosing between varied health plans. There is limited consideration in these studies, though, on how consumers define quality nursing care.

Research on consumers' perspectives of health care quality and what quality nursing care means to them will contribute to a better understanding of how the public views quality care and their expectations for care. Providers' perceptions of quality often differ from patients' perceptions. Consumer information about quality care lets providers know what is important to the public about their health care in general, their medical care, and their nursing care.

The expectations of consumers influence their satisfaction with care. Expectations for care have been defined differently in the literature. Some studies view patients' expectations as probabilities—judgments about the likelihood that a set of events will occur. Others view expectations as values—patients' desires about care expressed as perceived needs, wants, importance, standards, or entitlements. Whether patient expectations are considered as probabilities or values, an understanding of patient expectations is important because meeting these expectations may lead to greater satisfaction with care.

Whereas many studies have been done on patient satisfaction with nursing care, most of this research focuses on satisfaction with a specific health care encounter, such as a hospitalization or outpatient visit. Less is known about how people view quality care in general.

Adapted from: Oermann, M.H. (1999). Consumers' descriptions of quality health care. *Journal of Nursing Care Quality, 14*(1), 47–48. With permission © 1999, Aspen Publishers.

5. Follow the style manual or author guidelines to determine how to level the headings and position them in the manuscript, as well as other details for typing them.

6. Avoid abbreviations in headings, even if expanded earlier in the manuscript. Instead, the author should write out the term or phrase.

7. Use parallel grammatical structure for subheadings within a section.

 ## REVIEW BY OTHERS

After the author has revised the first draft of the manuscript, it can be sent to co-authors to read. Some authors also find it helpful to have colleagues review the content and organization of the paper.

| DISPLAY 9.3 | **Sample Document With Headings** |

CONSUMER VIEWS OF QUALITY CARE

An important area of current research focuses on providing quality information to consumers. Despite extensive research on defining and measuring the quality of health care, less attention has been given to consumers' perspectives of quality care. Most of the studies examine the type of information valuable in choosing among varied health plans. There is limited consideration in these studies, though, on how consumers define quality nursing care.

IMPORTANCE OF RESEARCH WITH CONSUMERS

Research on consumers' perspectives of health care quality and what quality nursing care means to them will contribute to a better understanding of how the public views quality care and their expectations for care. Providers' perceptions of quality often differ from patients' perceptions. Consumer information about quality care lets providers know what is important to the public about their health care in general, their medical care, and their nursing care.

RELATIONSHIP TO PATIENT SATISFACTION

The expectations of consumers influence their satisfaction with care. Expectations for care have been defined differently in the literature. Some studies view patients' expectations as probabilities—judgments about the likelihood that a set of events will occur. Others view expectations as values—patients' desires about care expressed as perceived needs, wants, importance, standards, or entitlements. Whether patient expectations are considered as probabilities or values, an understanding of patient expectations is important because meeting these expectations may lead to greater satisfaction with care.

Whereas many studies have been done on patient satisfaction with nursing care, most of this research focuses on satisfaction with a specific health care encounter, such as a hospitalization or outpatient visit. Less is known about how people view quality care in general.

Adapted from: Oermann, M.H. (1999). Consumers' descriptions of quality health care. *Journal of Nursing Care Quality, 14*(1), 47–48. With permission © 1999, Aspen Publishers.

Review by Co-Authors

When to send the draft to co-authors is a decision of the first author or whoever is responsible for organizing the preparation of the manuscript. Usually, co-authors are asked to critique a second or subsequent draft of the manuscript rather than the first draft. The first draft may not contain the essential content, and the lead author may find in revising the draft that a reorganization of the content is warranted. It usually is best for co-authors to read a draft that the lead author has revised for accuracy and structure. The lead author should clarify for contributors that the focus of their review is to evaluate the content and its organization, not writing style.

All co-authors should read at least one of the early drafts and suggest revisions or give approval of the draft (Huth, 1999). The final version of the paper must be read and approved by each co-author to meet the requirements for authorship, as described in earlier chapters. In some cases, if a co-author reads and approves one of the later drafts of the manuscript and is unable to read the final version, the co-author can give written permission to the lead author to submit the paper. This permission should be in writing, should indicate which draft was read and approved, and should state that the co-author authorizes the lead author to submit the manuscript without the co-author's final approval (Huth, 1999, p. 162).

Drafts should be numbered, dated, and labeled with the co-author's name to track revisions of the manuscript. If contributors are reading drafts of individual sections of the paper, this should be noted. As the lead author receives suggestions for revisions, these can be made in subsequent drafts. All versions of the manuscript should be kept by the lead author or individual organizing preparation of the paper in case the authors need to refer to them later.

Review by Colleagues

The author might ask colleagues to review and critique the manuscript. Often, colleagues can identify missing content, problems with the organization of the content, and areas in which the presentation of the information is unclear. Ideally, colleagues asked to the critique the manuscript at this point in the revision process have an understanding of the content. The goal of this revision is to improve the content and its organization, not the writing style; this should be made clear to persons asked to review the paper. The author then can acknowledge these individuals in the manuscript as long as they give written approval.

 ## REVISING WRITING STRUCTURE AND STYLE

Publication of the manuscript depends more on the substantive content than on writing style, but poorly written papers may influence the critique by peer reviewers and the editor and ultimately the acceptance decision. If similar papers are under review, the one that is well written is more likely to be accepted. Poor writing structure and style also may result in extensive revisions before the manuscript is accepted for publication. Therefore, the author should carefully edit the manuscript so that it is well written.

Huth (1999) identified five qualities of good scientific prose:

- Fluency: Correct sequence of thoughts and order of ideas; connecting paragraphs, sentences, and ideas in the manuscript
- Clarity: Clear structure of content, paragraphs with clear intent and limited to that intent, clear use of modifiers, unambiguous antecedents for pronouns, and correct verb tenses
- Accuracy: Correct choice of words to convey meaning and correct spelling of words
- Economy: Elimination of unneeded words, phrases, and sentences
- Grace: Writing without offending readers, such as avoiding gender stereotypes, dehumanizing words, jargon, and distracting words.

The following section provides a framework for revising the writing structure and style. The author should begin by editing paragraphs, then move to revising sentences, phrases, and words (Fig. 9-1). This system enables the author to edit broad elements of the paper first, then move to more specific ones. Otherwise, changes may be made in words, phrases, and sentences that need to be modified again when the paragraph is edited.

The following discussion is not intended to be an exhaustive list of points to consider when editing the draft to improve the writing. The discussion highlights some of the aspects that the author must check when editing the writing structure and style.

In these revisions, authors should continue to keep earlier versions of the paper for referral later, if needed. If authors are making their own revisions, the manuscript may be modified easily on the computer. Alternately, some authors prefer to print hard copies and revise the prose on the hard copy to avoid being distracted by word processing. If revisions are made first on the hard copy, the author might use proofreaders' marks to indicate changes. Appendix 2 includes a list of proofreaders' marks and an example of their use in revising a draft.

Revise Paragraphs

One way to begin is by first editing the paragraphs. In editing the paragraphs, the author should check the (1) length, (2) introductory sentence, (3) structure, and (4) transitions between paragraphs.

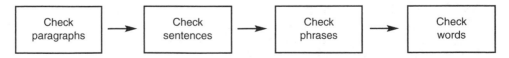

Figure 9-1. Scheme for revising writing structure and style.

Length

Paragraphs provide a means of discussing an area of similar content and presenting related details about that content; it is hard to imagine reading a paper without paragraphing. In a manuscript, paragraphs provide a strategy for moving from one idea to another through the paper. When the reader completes a paragraph and begins the following one, there is a sense of moving to a new idea or to different points about the content.

Excessively long paragraphs make it difficult for readers to keep track of ideas and are tiring to read. Therefore, Pearsall (1997) recommended paragraphing often and avoiding lengthy paragraphs. A paragraph that extends more than a typed page, double-spaced, probably is too long. Huth (1999) indicated that paragraphs more than 25 typed lines are likely to be too long.

Long paragraphs often can be divided into two smaller ones by identifying breaks in the flow of ideas or how details might be grouped together into separate paragraphs. For example, a lengthy paragraph on different addiction models might be divided into separate paragraphs, each describing one of the models. The initial paragraph in the sequence could specify the models discussed, listing them in the same order as explained in the paragraphs that follow.

Introductory Sentence

The first sentence of the paragraph introduces its topic and often is the transition from the preceding paragraph (Pearsall, 1997). In a paragraph that begins, "There are two major principles in evaluating a burn wound," the reader expects the paragraph to cover these two principles. The author should read the first sentence of each paragraph to determine if it adequately introduces the topic and content presented in the paragraph.

Structure

In editing the paragraph structure, the author is concerned with the sequence of ideas. As noted earlier, the beginning sentence introduces the content in the paragraph. The author then should confirm that there is a clear sequence of ideas developed from sentence to sentence through the paragraph.

Transitions Between Paragraphs

To develop ideas in the paper, paragraphs need to be linked to one another. Transitions lead readers from one section of the manuscript to the other (Sheridan & Dowdney, 1997). Readers should be able to track the main idea from the beginning of the paper to the end and follow the content from one paragraph to the next. To edit the transitions between paragraphs, the author should read the last sentence of a paragraph and first sentence of the next paragraph. Fondiller (1999) noted that when a paragraph "sounds like a new beginning," it needs revision (p. 86). Display 9.4 shows how paragraphs are connected so that a transition is formed between them and how ideas are developed by reading a sequence of paragraphs.

Revise Sentences

Next, the author reviews the length and structure of the sentences within each paragraph. Is each sentence clear? Does the sentence convey the meaning intended by the author? Are sentences too long? Are they too short? Are there any run-on sentences? Is there variety in how sentences are developed to maintain reader interest? Huth (1999) recommended varying the length and structure of sentences to avoid monotony.

Sentences link ideas to one another, providing a transition from preceding sentences and leading into the next sentence. Therefore, the author checks the flow of sentences throughout the manuscript. The writing also should keep the reader's interest.

In this stage of revision, the author also ensures that each sentence is grammatically correct: there should be subject–verb agreement (a singular subject with a singular verb and plural subject with a plural verb), and sentences should be punctuated correctly. Authors should check that parallel structure is used in sentences that contain a sequence of phrases or words. For example:

DISPLAY 9.4   Sample Paragraphing With Transitions

Evaluation fulfills two major roles in the classroom and clinical setting: formative and summative. Formative evaluation is feedback to learners about their progress in meeting the objectives and developing competencies for practice. It occurs throughout the instructional process and provides a basis for determining where further learning is needed.

Considering that the purpose of formative evaluation is to provide feedback on the progress being made in learning, formative evaluation typically is not graded. The teacher must remember that formative evaluation is designed to assess where further learning is needed.

Summative evaluation, on the other hand, is end-of-instruction evaluation designed to determine what the student has learned in the classroom and clinical setting. Summative evaluation provides information on the extent to which objectives were achieved, not on the progress of the learner in meeting them.

From Oermann, M.H., & Gaberson, K. (1998). *Evaluation and testing in nursing education* (pp. 4–5). New York: Springer. Reprinted with permission of Springer.

Original: Benefits of simulations are *learning* how to use equipment, *developing* ability to perform a procedure, and *to practice* complex technological skills in a laboratory environment rather than with actual patients.

Revised for parallel structure: Benefits of simulations are *learning* how to use equipment, *developing* ability to perform a procedure, and *practicing* complex technological skills in a laboratory environment rather than with actual patients.

Revise Words

In revising the sentences, the author likely made numerous changes in the words used to describe ideas and connect sentences. The focus of this last phase of editing the manuscript is to examine the words used in each sentence, if they convey the correct meaning, and if the writing is clear. For some authors, reading the manuscript out loud helps to identify where revisions are needed.

Some guidelines follow:

* Check the clarity of the writing. The goal is to write clearly, accurately, and concisely. Zilm (1998) emphasized that simple words have more impact than long, complex words.
* Check for misplaced modifiers. Often, this problem can be avoided if the modifying word, phrase, or clause is placed close to the word that it is modifying. In the first example, the modifier is misplaced; the patient has congestive heart failure, not the nurse.
  * Original: The patient was transferred to the home health nurse with congestive heart failure.
  * Revision: The patient *with congestive heart failure* was transferred to the home health nurse.
* Check the verb tenses so that they are consistent throughout the paper and the correct verb tense is used. The correct verb tense is needed so that readers know when the action occurred. For instance, in the first statement, the use of past tense indicates to the readers that the study was completed earlier and is presented for historical purposes.

  In 1993, Jones completed the first study on evaluating the effects of using the computer for teaching patients in clinics

If the study by Jones still is important, the author might revise the sentence using the present perfect tense and delete the date:

  Jones has completed a study on evaluating the effects of using the computer for teaching patients in clinics.

In referring to current studies, present tense may be used:

> Smith reports that computers are effective for teaching patients in clinics.

- Check that the words express the intended meaning and are used correctly in the sentence. For example:
    - ✔Among (general, common relations in a group of more than two) versus between (relation between two objects or one thing and several objects):

        The work to be done was divided *among* the three nurse managers.

        The work to be done was divided *between* the nurse manager and the clinical coordinator.

    - ✔Affect (verb meaning to influence) versus effect (noun, or when used as a verb, its meaning is to bring about change or to cause):

        Patients were *affected* positively by the intervention, reporting decreased pain and improved coping.

        The *effects* of the intervention were decreased pain and improved coping.

    - ✔Normal and abnormal; positive and negative (the findings and results of tests and examinations are normal, abnormal, positive, or negative, not the tests and examinations themselves):

        Incorrect: The physical examination given by the nurse practitioner was normal.

        Correct: The *findings* from the physical examination given by the nurse practitioner were normal.

    - ✔Which (relative pronoun used to introduce a nonessential clause) versus that (relative pronoun used to introduce a necessary clause):

        The patient should have a complete assessment, *which* is described in this article, when admitted to the hospital.

        The author should check *that* the statistics are reported correctly.

- Delete excessive and unnecessary words. Publishing is expensive, so the author should omit unneeded words and phrases. For example:

> *In order to* evaluate neck masses, a thorough and complete examination of the head and neck region should be performed by the nurse practitioner *using a systematic process.*

"In order to" is an unnecessary phrase that can be omitted while still preserving the meaning of the sentence. Similarly, examinations are done systemati-

TABLE 9.1

Revising Unnecessary Words

Unnecessary Words	More Concise
a decreased amount (number) of	less (fewer)
a number of	many, several
accounted for by the fact	because
along the lines of	similar, like
an adequate amount of	enough
as a consequence of	because of
as of this date	today
at a period of time when	when
at this point in time	now
by means of	with, by
consensus of opinion	consensus
due to the fact that	because
during the course of	during, while
fewer in number	fewer
for the purpose of	for, to
for the reason that	since, because
given an account of	describe
has been engaged in the study of	has studied
has the capability of	can
in a position to	can
in an effort to	to
in all cases	all, always
in close proximity to	near
in excess of	more than
in my opinion, I think	I think
in order to	to
in regard to	about
in the event that	if
in view of, in view of the fact that	because
it has been reported by Smith	Smith reported
it would appear that	apparently
make reference to	refer to
many in number	many
of great benefit	beneficial
on account of	because
on the basis of	because, from
prior to (in time)	before
regardless of the fact that	even though

(continued)

cally, so the phrase "using a systematic process" is not needed. By eliminating unnecessary words in this sentence, it reads:

> To evaluate neck masses, a thorough and complete examination of the head and neck region should be performed by the nurse practitioner.

Table 9.1 (p. 197) provides a list of unneeded words and phrases. The author also should check for adjectives and adverbs that are not essential to the sentence, such as "very" and "really." For example:

> The possibility of having a mass in the neck region may be *very* stressful to patients.

"Very" does not add to the meaning of the sentence and may be omitted. Another example is as follows:

> There was a *large* increase in the number of patients admitted to home care with the initiation of case management.

"Large" in this sentence is vague; it would be better to present the actual increase in numbers of patients admitted to home care within a particular time period.

* Check the antecedents of pronouns. When using pronouns, make it clear to which word they are referring. For example:

> Jones and Smith reported that patients learned effectively with videotapes. *They* were satisfied with the quality of the instruction.

In the second sentence, it is not clear to whom "they" refers: Is it Jones and Smith who were satisfied with the quality of the instruction or the patients?

TABLE 9.1	
Revising Unnecessary Words (CONTINUED)	
Unnecessary Words	**More Concise**
subsequent to	after
take into consideration	consider
the majority of, the vast majority of	most
with reference to	about
X-year period of time	X years

Adapted from: Day, R.A. (1998). *How to write and publish a scientific paper* (5th ed., pp. 238–243). Phoenix, AZ: Oryx Press; Huth, E.J. (1999). *Writing and publishing in medicine* (3rd ed., pp. 189–190). Baltimore: Williams & Wilkins; and Sheridan, D.R., & Dowdney, D.L. (1997). *How to write and publish articles in nursing* (2nd ed., p. 208). New York: Springer.

Ambiguity often results when sentences begin with "it" and "this," requiring readers to refer to the prior sentence. Authors are advised to check each pronoun for clarity.

- Check for spelling errors. The spell-checking function in word-processing programs identifies misspelled words, although medical and specialized terms often need to be checked by the author. The author also should be alert to words that are spelled correctly but misused in the sentence, for instance, principle versus principal. Only careful reading by the author, not the word-processing program, will locate these errors.

- Avoid gender bias in writing. To illustrate, references characterizing nurses as women and patients as men are stereotypes to be avoided. Often, this problem can be addressed by using the plural form. For example:
  - Original: The nurse begins teaching when *she* completes the initial assessment of learning needs.
  - Revised: Nurses begin teaching when *they* complete the initial assessment of learning needs.
  - Original: The patient should have an opportunity to choose *his* own treatment.
  - Revised: Patients should have the opportunity to choose *their* own treatments.

  In other situations, the author may modify the words to avoid reference to gender, for example, using committee chair or chairperson rather than chairman.

- Avoid impersonal writing.
  - Original: The diabetic should be taught about diet and medication.
  - Revised: The patient with diabetes should be taught about diet and medication.

- Use active voice (stating who or what the person is doing) versus passive voice (in which the subject is acted on). Sheridan and Dowdney (1997) indicated that overuse of passive voice makes writing awkward. For example:
  - Passive voice: The clinical guidelines were developed by the interdisciplinary team.
  - Active voice: The interdisciplinary team developed the clinical guidelines.

- Check capitalization of proper nouns and names of organization and institutions.

- Avoid using jargon and abbreviated terms such as "temp" and "lab." Jargon and abbreviations can be used in the drafts of the paper to capture the ideas for the manuscript but then need to be rewritten during the revision.
  - Original: The nurse *prepped* the patient for surgery after checking *lab* values.
  - Revised: The nurse *prepared* the patient for surgery after checking *laboratory* values.

Display 9.5 is a checklist for authors to use in revising their drafts for writing structure and style. As mentioned earlier, this discussion does not include all of the principles to consider in improving writing but highlights some important ones for the author to follow.

REVIEW SCIENTIFIC STYLE

Publications in nursing and health care often include abbreviations, symbols, measures, and other labels for presenting specialized content. Similar to for-

---

DISPLAY 9.5 **Checklist for Revising Writing Structure and Style**

✔ Ideas are sequenced clearly throughout the manuscript as a whole and in each section.
✔ Paragraphs focus on one topic and present details about it.
✔ Clear sequence of ideas is developed within paragraphs.
✔ Clear transitions exist between paragraphs.
✔ First sentence of paragraph introduces subject and provides transition from preceding paragraph.
✔ Paragraphs are of appropriate length.
✔ Sentences are written clearly and convey intended meaning.
✔ Sentences are of appropriate length.
✔ Variety is present in types of sentences and how they begin.
✔ Clear transitions exist between sentences.
✔ Words express intended meaning and are used correctly.
✔ Clear antecedents for pronouns are used.
✔ Modifiers are not misplaced.
✔ Excessive and unnecessary words are omitted.
✔ Stereotypes, impersonal writing, jargon, and abbreviated terms are avoided.
✔ Active voice is used.
✔ Grammar: Correct?
✔ Punctuation: Correct?
✔ Capitalization: Correct?
✔ Spelling: Correct?
✔ Writing keeps readers' interest.

mats for references, journals have their own style for reporting scientific information. This information may be provided in the journal guidelines, but usually the author refers to a style manual such as the *AMA Manual of Style: A Guide for Authors and Editors* (AMA, 1998) or the *Publication Manual of the American Psychological Association* (APA, 1994). In the revision of the manuscript, the author verifies the proper use of abbreviations, nomenclature, units of measure, numbers and percentages, and statistics. Display 9.6 summarizes these principles in the form of a checklist.

Abbreviations

An abbreviation is a shortened form of a word, such as U.S. for United States. An acronym is a word formed from the initial letters of words in a phrase, such as CINAHL formed from Cumulative Index to Nursing and Allied Health

---

DISPLAY 9.6   **Checklist for Scientific Style**

ABBREVIATIONS

☐ Expanded first time they are cited in text followed by initials in parentheses
☐ No abbreviations in title or abstract
☐ No author-invented abbreviations

NOMENCLATURE

☐ Standard nomenclature used

UNITS OF MEASURE

☐ SI used for measurements except for temperature, blood pressure, and time

NUMBERS AND PERCENTAGES

☐ Figures used for numbers 10 and above
☐ Figures used for statistics, fractions, decimals, and percentages
☐ Words used for numbers below 10 except when grouped with numbers 10 and above in the same sentence
☐ Words used for common fractions
☐ Words used if sentence, title, or heading begins with a number
☐ Percentage used when specific number not included

STATISTICS

☐ Statistical analysis and interpretations correct
☐ Data in text consistent with tables and figures
☐ Complete information reported with each statistic
☐ Accepted abbreviations and symbols used
☐ Statistics typed correctly

Literature. An acronym is pronounced as a word. An initialism is a name formed from the initials of an organization such as ANA for American Nurses Association (AMA, 1998). When writing a manuscript, the author can consider these together, all representing a type of abbreviation in writing.

Most journals discourage abbreviations in manuscripts because abbreviations commonly used in one specialty in nursing may not be understood by readers with different clinical backgrounds and experiences. The exceptions though are standard and approved abbreviations, such as those found in a style manual, and when words are repeated throughout a manuscript, for example, using CINAHL rather than Cumulative Index to Nursing and Allied Health Literature.

When abbreviations are used, the author writes out the words at their first citation in the manuscript followed by the initials in parentheses. Afterward, the initials can be used alone:

> Length of stay (LOS) decreased from 4.0 to 2.5 days after implementation of the critical pathway. With improved medication management, LOS decreased by an additional 1.2 days.

Abbreviations, though, should not be used in the title or abstract (Day, 1998). The reader should understand words and phrases in the title and abstract without referring to the text. This is particularly important in bibliographic databases that contain abstracts of articles; the abstract should be clear to individuals searching the database.

In the draft, the author should write out the words, then during the revision, add the abbreviations after the first citation. Otherwise, content might be reorganized, altering the first time the abbreviation is used in the manuscript. It also allows the author to keep a draft without abbreviations in case this information is needed later.

Nomenclature

For clinical papers, the author may need to refer to specific diseases, diagnostic tests, terminology, medications, and names for other entities. Nomenclature is the formulation of names to represent these entities. For example, the author might describe care of a patient with stage IV cancer, indicate that the patient had a grade 4 systolic murmur, report an Apgar score of 9 at 1 minute, and include the Po_2 value in a manuscript. Some symbols may be used without expanding them the first time cited in the paper, such as Po_2, whereas others should be written out the first time, such as positive end-expiratory pressure (PEEP). For medications, authors should use the nonproprietary (generic) name, which is the official name of the drug (AMA, 1998). Authors are not expected to remember these rules and instead should write out the terms in the first draft, then in the revision refer to the style manual for how to correctly cite them in the paper.

Units of Measure

The International System of Units (SI) is considered the universal measurement standard, providing uniformity in expressing measurements (AMA, 1998). It is a refinement of the metric system. Non-SI units used in papers are measurements for temperature, blood pressure, and time. The requirements for metric style are well established, so authors should be careful to check the style manual to ensure consistency.

Numbers and Percentages

There are several style requirements when reporting numbers and percentages. A few are summarized here, but again, the author is advised to check a style manual.

1. In general, use figures for numbers 10 and above, for example, 30 years old, 10 cm wide, 15% of the group, and 207 participants.
2. Use words for numbers less than 10, for example, "Subjects completed five instruments."
3. However, for numbers less than 10 that are grouped with numbers 10 and above in the same sentence or paragraph, use the figures. For example:
   In 4 of the 27 patients, acute pain was reported.
   The children's ages ranged from 2 to 11 years.
4. Use figures for statistics, fractions, decimals, and percentages, for example, $P = .04$, 5½ days, 0.25, and less than 8%.
5. Use words for common fractions, for example, one fourth.
6. If a sentence, title, or heading begins with a number, use words to represent the number, for example, "Twenty-four of the patients were discharged within 5 days of admission."

Percent means by the hundred; the word percent and symbol % are used with a specific number (AMA, 1998). Percentage is used when a number is not included. For example:

Eighty percent of the nurses had high levels of job satisfaction.
Pain was reported by 25% of the patients.
Of the 120 patients, 62 (51.7%) had improved scores on the posttest.
Anxiety was reported by a small percentage of the nursing students.

Statistics

Reporting statistics in research papers is described in Chapter 6. When revising the paper, the author should check carefully that the statistical analysis is correct, the data in the text are consistent with the tables and figures, and complete information is included when reporting the statistics. What constitutes complete information depends on the statistic reported, and the author should consult a style manual or statistics book for direction.

In reporting statistics, accepted abbreviations and symbols must be used. Common ones are listed in Appendix 1. Many statistical abbreviations, such as SD for standard deviation, are not expanded the first time cited in the text. Others, though, such as ANOVA, may be written out at the first mention in the text with the abbreviation in parentheses, depending on the style manual. The author should follow the guidelines specified in the style manual.

When checking the statistics,

1. Review the original statistical analysis to confirm that the statistics reported in the manuscript and interpretations are correct.
2. Compare the data and statistics reported in the text with the tables and figures.
3. Refer to the style manual or statistics book to ensure that complete information is presented with each statistic reported and the appropriate abbreviations and symbols are used and typed properly.
4. Use the statistical term, not the symbol, when referring to a statistic in the narrative. For example, instead of "The M score was 125," the text should read, "The mean score was 125."
5. Use an uppercase and italicized N for the number of subjects in the total sample (eg, $N = 206$). A lowercase, italicized n represents the number of subjects in a portion of the total sample. For example, "Group 1 included managers ($n = 32$) and staff ($n = 16$)."
6. Remember that statistical symbols are typeset in italic type but are underlined on the manuscript.

 SUMMARY

The goal in writing the first draft of the manuscript is to present the essential content in a logical order. With this objective in mind, the initial revisions of the draft focus on the content and how it is organized, not on grammar, punctuation, spelling, and writing style. There is no set number of drafts to write until satisfied with the content, although writing at least three drafts is likely.

If the author developed a working title, this can be reviewed first. The title should capture the purpose of the manuscript. In reviewing the abstract, the author examines if it adequately summarizes the purpose of the paper, indicating the most important content within the length allowed by the journal. For research manuscripts, the abstract should describe the study purpose and background, methods, and findings.

In reviewing the main body of the paper, the author begins by reading the introductory section. The key is to assess if the introduction explains the content covered in the paper and its importance to readers. After critiquing the introduction, the author then is ready to review the rest of the text. The author should reread the draft to determine if content is missing, if content can be omitted, and if there is repetitive content; to assess the organization or structure of the paper; and to determine the accuracy of the content. Unnecessary references should be deleted at this stage, and each table and figure should be reviewed to determine if it is essential to the paper.

Headings and subheadings emphasize the content covered in each section of the manuscript. They indicate the organization of the manuscript, provide transition from one topic to the next, inform readers of the content that follows, and suggest the importance of each subject area. In the revision stage, the author has the opportunity to add headings and subheadings to the manuscript.

After the first draft is revised, the author continues revising the drafts until satisfied with the content and its organization. Usually, co-authors are asked to critique a second or subsequent draft of the manuscript rather than the first draft. The final version of the paper must be read and approved by each co-author to meet the requirements for authorship.

Publication of the manuscript depends more on the substantive content than on writing style, but poorly written papers may influence the critique by peer reviewers and the editor and, ultimately, the acceptance decision. Therefore, the author must carefully edit the manuscript so that it is well written. The author can begin by editing paragraphs, then move to revising sentences, phrases, and words. This system enables the author to edit broad elements of the paper first, then move to specifics. In the revision of the manuscript, the author verifies the proper use of abbreviations, nomenclature, units of measure, numbers and percentages, and statistics. The chapter discusses some of the aspects of writing for the author to check when editing the writing structure and style.

REFERENCES

American Medical Association. (1998). *Manual of style: A guide for authors and editors* (9th ed.). Baltimore: Lippincott Williams & Wilkins.

American Psychological Association (APA). (1994). *Publication manual of the American Psychological Association* (4th ed.). Washington, DC: APA.

Black, J. (1995). Writing for publication: Advice to potential authors. *Plastic Surgical Nursing, 16*, 90–93.

Day, R.A. (1998). *How to write and publish a scientific paper* (5th ed.). Phoenix, AZ: Oryx Press.

Fondiller, S.H. (1999). *The writer's workbook* (2nd ed.). Sudbury, MA: Jones & Bartlett.

Huth, E.J. (1999). *Writing and publishing in medicine* (3rd ed.). Baltimore: Lippincott Williams & Wilkins.

McConnell, C.R. (1999). From idea to print: Writing for a professional journal. *Health Care Supervisor, 17*(3), 72–85.

Muscari, M.E. (1998). Do the write thing: Writing the clinically focused article. *Journal of Pediatric Health Care, 12,* 236–241.

Oermann, M.H. (1999a). Extensive writing projects: Tips for completing them on time. *Nurse Author & Editor, 9*(1), 8–10.

Oermann, M.H. (1999b). Writing for publication as an advanced practice nurse. *Nursing Connections, 12*(3), 5–13.

Pearsall, T.E. (1997). The elements of technical writing. Boston: Allyn & Bacon.

Sheridan, D.R., & Dowdney, D.L. (1997). *How to write and publish articles in nursing* (2nd ed.). New York: Springer.

Zilm, G. (1998). *The SMART way: An introduction to writing for nurses.* Toronto, Canada: Harcourt Brace & Company.

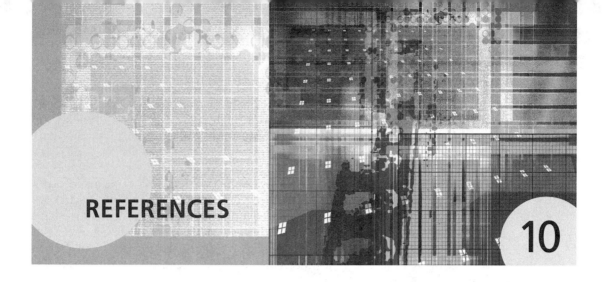

REFERENCES

Most papers written for publication in nursing include references. The references in the manuscript document the literature reviewed by the author in preparing the paper and provide support for its ideas. Chapter 5 discusses how to conduct and write a literature review for a manuscript. It describes the purposes of a literature review, bibliographic databases useful for literature reviews in nursing, selecting which databases to use, search strategies, analyzing and synthesizing the literature, and writing the literature review. The outcome of Chapter 5 is for authors to develop skill in conducting literature reviews for writing papers in nursing.

This chapter focuses on citing the references in the manuscript and preparing the reference list. Journals have different reference formats, and the author must prepare the references according to the journal guidelines. Most of these reference styles are based on either the name-year system or citation-sequence system. These two systems are discussed in the chapter, and examples are provided on how to cite references in the text and on the reference list itself using both systems. The author needs to consult a style manual for more information about preparing different types of references using each system.

REFERENCE STYLES

Journals differ in the styles they use for citations and references. Two of the reference styles widely used in nursing and health care journals are the name-year system and the citation-sequence system. In the name-year system, which is used in this book, the author's name and year of publication are used; this system sometimes is referred to as the "Harvard system" (Huth, 1999). The other reference format is the citation-sequence system, also known as the

"Vancouver system" (International Committee of Medical Journal Editors [ICMJE], 1997). Different journals have developed their own adaptations of these systems, so in preparing the citations in the text and the references, the author needs to carefully follow the information for authors page for the journal.

These reference styles include guidelines for citations and references. A "citation" is the documentation of the work in the text. The citation informs the readers that the statement or idea in the text was developed by the authors cited. In some styles, the citations are documented by author surname and year of publication, allowing readers to find the complete reference on the alphabetized list at the end of the manuscript. Other formats use a number to denote citations in text; the number corresponds to a publication on the reference list.

The reference list at the end of the manuscript documents the publications reviewed by the author in preparation of the paper and enables readers to retrieve them for their own work. A reference list cites the resources actually used in preparing the manuscript, whereas a bibliography includes other publications and information related to the content of the paper. The bibliography provides additional readings about the topic not cited in the manuscript. Most journals require reference lists, not bibliographies, although the author might prepare a bibliography for other writing projects.

References are placed at the end of the paper, after the text and before the tables and figures. All references cited in the text should be on the reference list, and all of the references in the list should be cited in the text. The author is responsible verifying this.

Because the reference list allows others to retrieve the references, information about each publication must be complete and accurate. Although there are numerous variations of reference formats, references to journals contain the following information:

- Authors' surnames and initials
- Year of publication
- Title of article (and subtitle)
- Name of journal
- Volume number
- Issue number or month if journal is paginated by issue
- Inclusive page numbers.

References to books contain the following information:

- Authors' surnames and initials
- Year of copyright
- Book title (and subtitle)

- Volume number and title if there is more than one volume
- Edition number (except when referencing a first edition)
- Place of publication
- Name of publisher.

When referring to a chapter in a book, the reference also includes the following:

- Chapter authors' surnames and initials
- Chapter title
- Inclusive page numbers of chapter.

There are specific formats for preparing references on articles in journals, books, book chapters, technical reports, proceedings of meetings and conferences, master's theses and doctoral dissertations, unpublished materials, audiovisual media, and electronic media. Providing examples of each of these formats is beyond the scope of this book, so the author guidelines of the journal or a style manual should be consulted.

The author guidelines either provide examples of how to prepare each type of reference or indicate the reference style to be used for manuscript preparation. For instance, the author guidelines for the *Western Journal of Nursing Research* direct authors to use the fourth edition of the *Publication Manual of the American Psychological Association* (APA, 1994). *Applied Nursing Research* uses APA style, and the information page for authors also provides examples on preparing references. Manuscripts written for *Nurse Practitioner* and *Journal of Nursing Care Quality* conform to *The Chicago Manual of Style* (1993). *Cancer Nursing* uses the citation-sequence system, where references are numbered consecutively according to the order in which they appear in the text. For the *Journal of Nursing Administration,* references are prepared according to the *American Medical Association Manual of Style* (AMA, 1998).

As can be seen in these examples, authors cannot assume that the journal for submission uses a particular reference style just because the author has used it in the past. Authors must prepare references according to the style specified by the journal (Oermann, 1999). If the manuscript is rejected and then sent to a different journal, the author is responsible for revising the citations and references to be consistent with that journal's style.

Name-Year System: Citations

In the name-year system, citations in the text include the authors' names, and year of publication in parentheses. The surname of the author and publication date are placed next to the statement being referenced:

> Smith (2000) found a significant relationship between student stress in the clinical setting and performance.
>
> A significant relationship was found between student stress in the clinical setting and performance (Smith, 2000).

Once the reference is cited in a paragraph, subsequent references in that same paragraph do not have to include the date of publication. For example:

> Smith (2000) found a significant relationship between student stress in the clinical setting and performance. The higher the level of stress, the lower the performance ratings. Smith also found differences in stress. . . .

For publications by multiple authors, different principles are followed for citing author names in the text. When the publication has two authors, both names are included each time the reference is cited in the text:

> Smith and Jones (2000) found a significant relationship between student stress in the clinical setting and performance.
>
> A significant relationship was found between student stress in the clinical setting and performance (Smith & Jones, 2000).

When there are three to five authors, the names are included the first time that the reference occurs in the text, but for subsequent citations, only the name of the first author is included followed by "et al." and the year published (APA, 1994). For example:

> Smith, Jones, Kaelig, Brown, and Dowd (2000) reported that... [first citation in text].
>
> Smith et al. (2000) reported that . . . [subsequent citations].

For references with more than six authors, only the surname of the first author is cited followed by "et al." (APA, 1994). In the reference list, though, all names are provided. When using "et al" (which means "and others"), only the surname of the first author is included, without a comma after the name and with a period after "al."

If the citation refers to a specific part of the original work, such as a quotation or statement on a particular page, then the page number also is included in the citation. An example follows:

> (Smith, 2000, p. 24).

Name-Year System: References

In the name-year system, the references are listed at the end of the manuscript in alphabetical order based on the surname of the first author. The year of publication, in parentheses, follows the last author name cited with the reference. When there is more than one reference by the same person, they are arranged by year of publication with the earliest listed first (APA, 1994). An example follows:

Basco, S., Gumbel, A.C., & Davies, R. (1995)

Jones, T.B. (1999)

Mathews, A.M. (1998)

Mathews, A.M., & Coleman, T. Z. (1997)

Smith, J.B. (1999)

Smith, J.B. (2000).

If there is more than one reference by an author or by the same two or more authors in identical order, published in the same year, these would be arranged alphabetically by title (APA, 1994, p. 179). Lowercase letters are placed after the year of publication to differentiate the citations. For example:

Smith, J.B., & Thompson, M. (2000a). Behavioral....

Smith, J.B., & Thompson, M. (2000b). Stress....

The APA *Publication Manual* provides detailed information about preparing references using the name-year system. Some journals use a variation of this system by listing the references in alphabetical order and then numbering them. These numbers are used for the citations in the text rather than the name and year of publication.

Display 10.1 presents sample references prepared according to the APA *Publication Manual*, which uses the name-year system, and the Uniform Requirements for Manuscripts Submitted to Biomedical Journals (ICMJE, 1997), which uses the citation-sequence system. These examples do not show every type of reference that could be cited in a paper, but they demonstrate the differences between the two formats.

Citation-Sequence System: Citations

Many journals use the citation-sequence system specified in the Uniform Requirements or use some adaptation of the system. The *American Medical Association Manual of Style* provides detailed information about preparing references with this system.

In the citation-sequence system, citations in the text, tables, and figures are denoted using Arabic numerals and are numbered consecutively. In the Uniform Requirements, the numerals are placed in parentheses, for example:

. . . developed and evaluated the clinical guidelines.(1-3)

DISPLAY 10.1	Name–Year and Citation–Sequence Systems

NAME–YEAR SYSTEM: AMERICAN PSYCHOLOGICAL ASSOCIATION REFERENCE FORMAT

Journal Article

Biel, M., Eastwood, J.A., Muenzen, P., & Greenberg, S. (1999). Evolving trends in critical care nursing practice: Results of a certification role delineation study. *American Journal of Critical Care, 8,* 285-290.

Journal Article With More Than Six Authors

Dunn, S.V., Lawson, D., Robertson, S., Underwood, M., Clark, R., Valentine, T., Walker, N., Wilson-Row, C., Crowder, K., & Herewane, D. (2000). The development of competency standards for specialist critical care nurses. *Journal of Advanced Nursing, 31,* 339-346.

Article in Journal Paginated by Issue

Kennedy-Schwarz, J. (2000). Pain management: A moral imperative. *American Journal of Nursing, 100*(8), 49-50.

Article in Journal With No Author Given

A new code of ethics for nurses. ANA's Code of Ethics Project Task Force. (2000). *American Journal of Nursing, 100*(7), 69-72.

Article With Organization as Author

American Association of Colleges of Nursing. (2000). Distance technology in nursing education: Assessing a new frontier. *Journal of Professional Nursing, 16,* 116-122.

Book by Author

Oermann, M.H., & Gaberson, K. (1998). *Evaluation and testing in nursing education.* New York: Springer.

Book by Editor:

Kovner, A.R., & Jonas, S. (Eds.). (1999). *Jonas and Kovner's health care delivery in the United States* (6th ed.). New York: Springer.

Chapter in Book

Weitzman, B.C. (1999). Improving quality of care. In A.R. Kovner & S. Jonas (Eds.), *Jonas and Kovner's health care delivery in the United States* (6th ed., pp. 370-400). New York: Springer.

Electronic Document

Certification. (2000). NursingCenter.com. Retrieved September 3, 2000, http://www.nursingcenter.com/ career/certification.cfm.

CITATION–SEQUENCE SYSTEM: UNIFORM REQUIREMENTS FOR MANUSCRIPTS SUBMITTED TO BIOMEDICAL JOURNALS

Journal Article

Biel M, Eastwood JA, Muenzen P, Greenberg S. Evolving trends in critical care nursing practice: results of a certification role delineation study. Am J Crit Care 1999;8:285-90.

(continued)

Journal Article With More Than Six Authors

Dunn SV, Lawson D, Robertson S, Underwood M, Clark R, Valentine T, et al. The development of competency standards for specialist critical care nurses. J Adv Nurs 2000;31:339-46.

Article in Journal Paginated by Issue

Kennedy-Schwarz J. Pain management: a moral imperative. Am J Nurs 2000;100(8):49-50.

Article in Journal With No Author Given

A new code of ethics for nurses. ANA's Code of Ethics Project Task Force. Am J Nurs 2000;100(7):69-72.

Article With Organization as Author

American Association of Colleges of Nursing. Distance technology in nursing education: assessing a new frontier. J Prof Nurs 2000;16:116-22.

Book by Author

Oermann MH, Gaberson K. Evaluation and testing in nursing education. New York: Springer; 1998.

Book by Editor

Kovner AR, Jonas S, editors. Jonas and Kovner's health care delivery in the United States. 6th ed. New York: Springer; 1999.

Chapter in Book

Weitzman BC. Improving quality of care. In: Kovner AR, Jonas, S, editors. Jonas and Kovner's health care delivery in the United States. 6th ed. New York: Springer; 1999. pp. 370-400.

Electronic Document

Certification. NursingCenter.com Web site. Available at: http://www.nursingcenter.com/career/certification.cfm. Accessed September 3, 2000.

In the *American Medical Association Manual of Style,* superscript numerals are used instead of numerals in parentheses. For formats using superscripts, the superscript numeral is placed outside of the periods and commas and inside colons and semicolons. When more than two references are cited, a hyphen is used to join the first and last number of the series (AMA, 1998, p. 30). Two examples follow:

> . . . examined by other researchers.[2-5]

> The teacher can prepare different types of objective test items for the course[7]: true-false, multiple choice. . . .

One advantage of using the citation-sequence system is that the numbered citations do not interrupt the text and flow of ideas, as sometimes occurs with the name-year system. A long list of references cited within one sentence may require the reader to skip over several lines of references to return to the text; even a few references cited together may be distracting (Day, 1998).

Citation-Sequence System: References

In the citation-sequence system, references at the end of the manuscript are numbered consecutively in the order in which they are first cited in the text (ICMJE, 1997). If the author guidelines specify that references should be prepared using the uniform requirements, they can be found at *http://www.ama-assn.org/public/peer/wame/uniform.htm* and also at *http://www.icmje.org*. The AMA reference format is described in the *American Medical Association Manual of Style*.

According to the Uniform Requirements and AMA style, the journal titles are abbreviated, and the year of publication follows the journal title, which differs from APA style. The titles of journals are abbreviated according to the style used in *Index Medicus*. If the author is unsure how to abbreviate the title, the author can find this information in the *List of Journals Indexed in Index Medicus* available through the National Library of Medicine at *http://www.nlm.nih.gov/tsd/serials/lji.html*.

In preparing the draft, citations in the text should be indicated by the author's name and publication date rather than numbered. Otherwise, as revisions are made in the draft and references are reordered, these numbers will change. The citations should be numbered in the final version of the paper.

The references for the following citation are prepared using the Uniform Requirements style. Other examples are presented in Display 10.1. Because of the many variations to the citation-sequence system, the author needs to follow the journal guidelines.

Citation: Whereas varied definitions of outcomes have been proposed, outcomes, in general, are the end results of a treatment or intervention.(1,2) While some outcomes are the result of specific nursing interventions, many other outcomes are achieved because of the multiple disciplines involved in the patient's care.(3)

References
1. Huber DL, Oermann MH. The evolution of outcomes management. In: Blancett SS, Flarey DL, editors. Health care outcomes: collaborative, path-based approaches. Gaithersburg, MD: Aspen; 1998. pp. 3-12.
2. Marek KD. Measuring the effectiveness of nursing care. Outcomes Manag Nurs Pract 1997;1:8-12.
3. Jones KR, Jennings BM, Moritz P, Moss MT. Policy issues associated with analyzing outcomes of care. Image J Nurs Sch 1997;29:261-7.

ELECTRONIC REFERENCE FORMATS

The proliferation of electronic information resources continues, and authors need to follow the style manual for citing these references. For questions about electronic references not covered in the style manuals, the author can refer to the selected Internet resources listed in Display 10.2.

The *Publication Manual of the American Psychological Association* includes a section on electronic reference formats, and additional information with examples is available at: *http://www.apa.org/journals/webref.html*. In general, when using APA style, the citation for a Web document follows a format similar to that for print, with some information added about the location of the site and when it was accessed. For example, the citation for the Web page on the APA electronic reference formats is as follows:

> *Electronic reference formats recommended by the American Psychological Association.* (2000, August 22). Washington, DC: American Psychological Association. Retrieved June 12, 2001, from the World Wide Web: http://www.apa.org/journals/webref.html.

When citing an entire Web site rather than a specific document on the site, the APA indicates that it is sufficient to give the address of the site in the text. No reference is needed on the reference list (APA, 2000). For example, "*Quick Checks for Quality* is a good consumer resource on quality health care (*http://www.ahcpr.gov/consumer/quick.htm*)." With the APA style, this resource would not be included on the reference list.

The *American Medical Association Manual of Style* provides guidelines for many types of electronic citations including software, on-line journals, CD-ROM, databases, Web sites, and email. When both print and electronic versions of the same document are available, authors cite the version that they used when preparing the manuscript. An example of a citation based on the *American Medical Association Manual of Style* for a Web document is as follows:

> Agency for Healthcare Research and Quality. Quick checks for quality: Choosing quality health care. Available at: http://www.ahcpr.gov/consumer/quick.htm. Accessed September 2, 2000.

The author should know the type of information required for the reference so that it can be recorded when the materials are accessed. When authors are completing their own searches, they can copy the URL and other information from the Web page that will be needed for the reference. The page even can be printed. Day (1998) recommends printing a hard copy of the Web page with the URL as an archived reference. Because of the rapid changes on the Web, the author should check the reference before submitting the paper to the journal and again when reviewing the page proofs to validate the URL and other information.

Internet Resources for Citing Electronic References

Electronic Reference Formats Recommended by the American Psychological Association.
Describes how to cite various electronic references with examples of each.
http://www.apa.org/elecref.html

Online! A Reference Guide to Using Internet Resources
Describes and provides examples of electronic reference formats for APA, MLA, Chicago, CBE, and other styles.
http://www.bedfordstmartins.com/online/citex.html

World Association of Medical Editors
Contains Uniform Requirements for Manuscripts Submitted to Biomedical Journals (ICMJE, 1997). Includes how to reference electronic material with examples.
http://www.ama-assn.org/public/peer/wame/uniform.html

MLA Style: Documenting Sources from the World Wide Web
Provides guidelines from the Modern Language Association (MLA) for documenting on-line references and includes examples.
http://www.mla.org/ (in section on frequently asked questions)

Electronic Sources: MLA Style of Citation
Describes and provides examples of electronic reference formats using MLA style.
http://www.bedfordstmartins.com/online/citex.html

International Organization for Standardization (ISO)
Worldwide federation of organizations and groups (non-governmental) to promote development of standards. Has developed standards for bibliographic references including electronic documents.
http://www.iso.ch/infoe/intro.html

International Federation of Library Associations and Institutions
Includes a list of style guides and resources for citing electronic references. Specifies data elements and their prescribed order in bibliographic references to electronic documents. Also includes examples.

 BIBLIOGRAPHIC MANAGEMENT SOFTWARE

Bibliographic management software such as EndNote, Reference Manager, and ProCite (ISI Research Soft, 2000) allows the author to search on-line bibliographic databases, store records, organize references in a database, and create reference lists automatically. They also enable the author to format manuscripts complete with citations and references for hundreds of reference styles. If the author decides later to submit the manuscript to another publication that uses a different reference style, the software automatically reformats the citations and references. This avoids retyping them. If using this software, the author needs to select the style that is required by the journal, making it easier to prepare the citations and references.

VERIFYING REFERENCES

Being careful to prepare accurate references cannot be overemphasized. Common errors that can occur with reference lists are (1) mistakes in the information provided in the reference, (2) errors in matching the citation with the correct reference, (3) failure to include all of the information needed with the reference, and (4) use of incorrect reference style. Authors can avoid these problems if they take time to review their references before submitting the manuscript (Brooks-Brunn, 1998).

The author should verify the accuracy of each reference against the original document, paying particular attention to the spelling of authors' names, initials, order of names, title of the document and publication in which it appears, and publication data. Book titles should be taken from the title page, not the cover, because sometimes titles are abbreviated on the cover (Zilm, 1998).

In reviewing the paper, the author should check that each citation is placed properly in the text and that the name or number corresponds with the correct reference at the end of the manuscript. In the name-year system, the spelling of authors' names and the year of publication cited in the text should be identical to the reference list, and references should be alphabetized correctly. In the citation-sequence system, the author should check that the reference number in the text matches the correct reference on the list at the end of the paper.

Once the information is verified, the author can check that all of the data are included in the reference, depending on the style, and the reference format is correct. Display 10.3 provides a checklist for verifying the references.

 ## SUMMARY

Journals differ in the styles used for citations and references. A citation is the documentation of the work in the text. The citation informs the readers that the statement or idea in the text was developed by the authors cited. A reference list includes the resources used in preparing the manuscript, whereas a bibliography provides additional readings about the topic not cited in the manuscript. Most journals require reference lists, not bibliographies.

Two of the reference styles widely used in nursing and health care journals are the name-year system and the citation-sequence system. In the name-year system, citations in the text include the author's name and year of publication in parentheses. References are listed at the end of the manuscript in alphabetical order based on the surname of the first author.

In the citation-sequence system, citations in the text are denoted using Arabic numerals (in parentheses or superscript) and are numbered consecutively. References are listed and numbered at the end of the manuscript according to

DISPLAY 10.3	**Checklist for Verifying References**

✔ Spelling of authors' names and year of publication in text with spelling and year in reference list

✔ Number of citation in text with correct reference

✔ Spelling of authors' names and verify accuracy of initials

✔ Order of authors' names listed with reference and if all names are included

✔ Date of publication

✔ Accuracy of title of document (eg, title of article, chapter, report)

✔ Accuracy of title of publication in which document appears (eg, journal title, book title)

✔ Abbreviation of journal title if relevant

✔ Accuracy of volume number, issue number if journal is paginated by issue, page numbers

✔ Capitalization

✔ Reference format

✔ Order of references

the order of citation in the text. Examples of these reference formats are provided. Journals use many adaptations of these systems, so in preparing the citations in the text and the references, the author needs to carefully follow the journal guidelines.

The proliferation of electronic information resources continues, and authors need to follow the style manual for how to cite these as references. Guidelines available on the Internet for documenting electronic references are provided as additional resources for the author to consult.

Being careful to prepare accurate references cannot be overemphasized. The errors made in reference lists can be avoided by verifying the reference with the original document and matching the citations in the text with the reference list. In the name-year system, the spelling of authors' names and the year of publication cited in the text should be identical to the reference list, and references should be alphabetized correctly. In the citation-sequence system, the author should check that the reference number cited in the text matches the correct reference at the end of the paper.

If using bibliographic management software, the author can select the reference style required by the journal. The citations and references then are prepared according to this style.

REFERENCES

American Medical Association. (1998). *Manual of style: A guide for authors and editors* (9th ed.). Baltimore: Lippincott Williams & Wilkins.

American Psychological Association (APA). (1994). *Publication manual of the American Psychological Association* (4th ed.). Washington, DC: APA.

American Psychological Association (APA). (2000). Electronic reference formats recommended by the American Psychological Association. [On-line]. Available: *http://www.apa.org/journals/webref.html*. Accessed June 11, 2001.

Brooks-Brunn, J.A. (1998). How and when to reference. *Nurse Author and Editor, 8*(2), 1–4.

The Chicago manual of style (14th ed.). (1993). Chicago: The University of Chicago Press.

Day, R.A. (1998). *How to write and publish a scientific paper* (5th ed.). Phoenix, AZ: Oryx Press.

Huth, E.J. (1999). *Writing and publishing in medicine* (3rd ed.). Baltimore: Lippincott Williams & Wilkins.

International Committee of Medical Journal Editors. (1997). Uniform requirements for manuscripts submitted to biomedical journals. *Annals of Internal Medicine, 126*, 36–47 Also available at *http://www.icmje.org/*

ISI Research Soft. (2000). Software to simplify your research. [On-line]. Available: *http://www.risinc.com*. Accessed June 16, 2000.

Oermann, M.H. (1999). Writing for publication as an advanced practice nurse. *Nursing Connections, 12*(3), 5–13.

Zilm, G. (1998). *The SMART way: An introduction to writing for nurses*. Toronto, Canada: Harcourt Brace & Company.

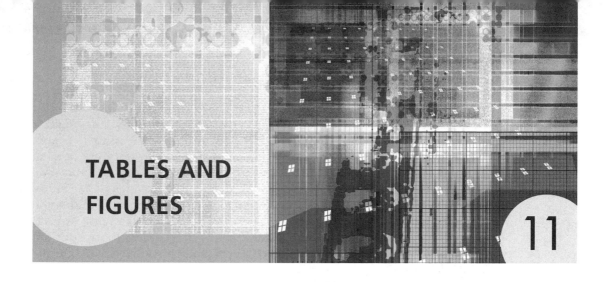

TABLES AND FIGURES

11

Tables are essential when the author needs to report detailed information and numeric values. It is often clearer and more efficient to develop a table than to present the information in the text. Figures such as graphs and charts are valuable for demonstrating trends and patterns. For some manuscripts, the author may include an illustration of a new procedure or equipment, or a photograph of a patient. Not every manuscript, though, needs tables and figures, and whether to include them is a decision made during the drafting phase of writing the paper. This chapter provides guidelines for deciding when to prepare tables and figures and how to develop them.

 ## NUMBER OF TABLES AND FIGURES

In writing the draft, the author needs to know the maximum number of tables and figures allowed. With this information, the author can avoid developing too many tables and figures for the length of the manuscript and specifications of the journal. It is helpful to prepare a draft of each table and figure as the manuscript is being written to confirm that the essential data are presented. The author can format these later, when the manuscript is revised.

Many journals limit the number—often to three—of tables and figures submitted with a manuscript. If the author guidelines do not specify the limit for tables and figures, the author can review current issues of the journal for the average number of tables and figures per article. As a general rule, Huth (1999) suggested that authors prepare one table or figure per 1000 words of text (p. 140).

TABLES

Tables are an effective way of presenting detailed and complex information succinctly and clearly. Tables should be used when the author wants to report exact values, present a large amount of information, display different quantitative values simultaneously, and show relationships among data. For research articles, tables are valuable for presenting the findings of the study with statistical results. In a table, the author can compare groups and show how differences across the groups were analyzed with accompanying results.

Tables also are valuable for emphasizing important information from the text. They can be used to highlight key concepts and focus attention on critical points discussed in the paper.

Tables present detailed information that supplements and supports the text without duplicating it. In the text, the author can discuss main findings from the table and highlight key points for readers to look for in the table. As an example, using the data from Display 11.2, a statement in text might be as follows:

> Of the 150 registered nurses, most (122, 81.3%) were in classifications II and III (Table 1).

Additional information about the number of nurses in each classification is available in the table, which avoids duplicating the text.

While tables support the text, they should be clear enough to "stand alone." Sufficient information should be included in the table for readers to understand it without referring to the text for an explanation. In revising the manuscript, the author should reread each table to ensure that it is an integral part of the text yet clear enough to be understood without reference to the text.

The data in tables should be accurate and consistent with the information reported in the text. To check this, the author can place each table next to the pages in the text where it is referenced and compare them for accuracy and consistency. If more than one table is used, they should be considered as a sequence with some relationship to one another (Huth, 1999).

Types of Tables

Authors can include various types of tables in a manuscript.

Tabulation

A tabulation is a short, informal table in the text that sets off the content from the text (American Medical Association [AMA], 1998). Tabulations usually contain only one or two columns, which are not placed within a formal table structure but instead are developed as part of the text (Display 11.1).

DISPLAY 11.1	In-Text Tabulation

The nursing process is a systematic way of collecting and analyzing patient data, identifying problems of patients, planning and implementing care, and evaluating its effectiveness. The five phases of the nursing process are as follows:

Phases	Definition
Assessment	Problem recognition and collection of data
Diagnoses	Data analysis and statement of nursing diagnoses
Plan	Setting priorities, developing goals, selecting interventions
Implementation	Carrying out nursing actions
Evaluation	Evaluating outcomes of care

The nursing process requires critical thinking, clinical judgment, and decision-making abilities. These cognitive abilities enable the nurse to consider alternate possibilities and evaluate options before making clinical decisions.

Traditional Table

A traditional or formal table contains information arranged in columns and rows. It is used to present quantitative data, statistical results, and detailed information. Most of the examples in this chapter are traditional tables. Each table has a title, headings to explain the columns and rows, and lines (called rules) that visually organize the data for the reader. Displays 11.2 and 11.3, Tables 11.2 to 11.4, and Figure 11-1 are examples of traditional tables.

Word Table

Word or text tables use words, phrases, and sentences, usually in lists, to describe the topic, highlight key points, and provide additional details to support the text. Similar to tables that present numerical data, word tables convey information that helps readers understand the content but is too detailed to be included in the text. For example, a table may be developed for a paper on care of the burn patient that lists potential patient problems, data to collect in an assessment with related laboratory tests, and interventions for each problem. Tables such as these, similar to ones that report quantitative data, should not be developed if the information can be presented clearly and concisely in the text. Table 11.1 is an example of a word table.

Use of Tables

In planning the manuscript, the author determines what information should be reported and then decides if this information is best communicated in a

TABLE 11.1

Word Table

Table 1: Phases of Nursing Process

Phase	Definition
Assessment	Recognizing problems and collecting data
Diagnosis	Analyzing data and identifying nursing diagnoses
Plan	Setting priorities, developing goals, selecting interventions
Implementation	Carrying out nursing interventions
Evaluation	Evaluating outcomes of care

table or in the text. There are two general principles for using tables in a manuscript.

First, do not use tables when the information can be reported instead in the text. Authors sometimes develop tables with information that could be presented easily in the text. When this is the case, a table should not be used. Readers may have difficulty following the data when numerous tables are used and may lose track of the message (American Psychological Association [APA], 1994). Using too many tables "breaks up" the text, and tables and figures are expensive to produce in a publication. Therefore, authors should use them wisely.

An example of this principle can be seen in Display 11.2. The information in Display 11.2 is presented in the form of a table and as text. Because the

DISPLAY 11.2 **Presenting Information in Table and as Text: Text Preferred**

AS TABLE

Table 1: Classifications of Registered Nurses

Classification	n (%)
I	28 (18.7)
II	56 (37.3)
III	66 (44.0)

AS TEXT

Of the 150 registered nurses, 28 (18.7%) were in classification I, 56 (37.3%) were in classification II, and the remaining nurses (n = 66, 44.0%) were in classification III.

information can be conveyed easily and concisely in the text, a table should not be developed.

Second, tables should be used when the author needs to report a large amount of data and exact numbers. Tables are an efficient way of presenting detailed information in a small amount of space and facilitating the comparison of information. Display 11.3 presents data in two ways: as a table and in the text. In contrast to the previous example, these data are best reported in the form of a table. They are too detailed for readers to follow in the text, limiting the ability to draw comparisons between the groups. Another example is Table 11.2. The correlations reported in this table are too extensive to include in the text, and the table provides a way to present all correlations—significant and insignificant—in one place.

Guidelines for Constructing Tables

The content in tables must be arranged logically and clearly so that readers can understand it and use it to easily locate specific data. In drafting the manuscript, the author plans what information is to be reported in the text and in tables. The next decision is how to best organize the information to make it clear to readers. Most tables are read first from left to right (horizontally), then from top to bottom (vertically) (AMA, 1998, p. 54). The author should remember this when deciding how to place data in a table. When the table is

---

DISPLAY 11.3   **Presenting Information in Table and as Text: Table Preferred**

AS TABLE

Table 1: Differences in Importance Ratings Between Men and Women

Importance Ratings	Men M (SD)	Women M (SD)	t
Able to call RN with questions	4.23 (.93)	4.92 (.95)	2.76*
Have RN teach illness, medications, treatment options	4.47 (.79)	4.40 (.90)	.568
Have RN teach health promotion	4.35 (.90)	4.00 (1.1)	2.51*

*$P < .01$

AS TEXT

Being able to call a registered nurse (RN) with questions after the clinic visit was more important to women ($M = 4.92$, $SD = .95$) than it was to men ($M = 4.23$, $SD = .93$) ($t = 2.76$, $df = 230$, $P < .01$). Teaching by the RN about the illness, medication, and treatments was equally important to men ($M = 4.47$, $SD = .79$) and women ($M = 4.40$, $SD = .90$) ($t = .568$, $df = 230$, $P = .57$). Health promotion teaching by an RN was more important to men ($M = 4.35$, $SD = .90$) than to women ($M = 4.00$, $SD = 1.1$) ($t = 2.51$, $df = 230$, $P < .01$).

TABLE 11.2

Sample Correlations Table

Table 1: Correlations of Quality Health Care Scores With Health Status

SF-36	Medical Care	Teaching by Nurse	Provider Competence	Choice of Provider	Nurse–Patient Interaction	Convenience of Appointments
Physical functioning	.124	−.057	.036	.113	−.049	−.150*
Role limitations (physical)	−.024	−.034	−.004	.106	−.132*	−.049
Pain	.082	−.009	−.023	.053	−.033	−.042
Vitality	.059	−.069	−.058	.127	−.130	−.089
Social functioning	.093	−.061	−.038	−.021	−.146*	−.126
Role limitations (emotional)	.065	−.161*	.001	.051	.022	−.024
Mental health	.127	−.160*	.016	.005	−.085	−.096
General health	.050	−.274**	.034	.144*	−.058	−.162*

$*p < .05, **p < .01$
Adapted from: Oermann, M.H., & Templin, T. (2000). Important attributes of quality health care: Consumer perspectives. *Journal of Nursing Scholarship, 32,* 170. Reprinted by permission of Sigma Theta Tau.

intended to compare groups or make before-and-after comparisons, it should be constructed so that readers can review the data horizontally, across the table. In Display 11.3, readers can compare scores for men and women on each of the three importance items by reading the scores horizontally.

Tables contain five major parts: title, body of the table, column headings, row headings, and footnotes (Fig. 11-1). This chapter provides general guidelines about how to construct tables; for further details, the author is directed to a style manual such as the *Publication Manual of the American Psychological Association* (APA, 1994) and the *American Medical Association Manual of Style: A Guide for Authors and Editors* (AMA, 1998).

Title

Every table needs a title. The title should be short, should describe the content in the table, and should be written as a phrase rather than as a sentence. The word "table" and its number are part of the title. In some style manuals, such as the AMA *Manual of Style*, the entire title is placed on one line (example 1). In other styles, such as the *Publication Manual of the American Psychological Association*, two lines are used and the title is underlined (example 2):

Example 1: Table 1. Classifications of Registered Nurses

Example 2: Table 1

Classifications of Registered Nurses

TABLE 1

Correlations of Quality Nursing Care Scores With Health Status

SF-36	Teaching by nurse	Nurse competence	Nurse–patient interaction
Physical functioning	−.057	.036	−.049
Role limitations (physical)	−.034	−.004	−.132*
Pain	−.009	−.023	−.033
Vitality	−.069	−.058	−.130
Social functioning	−.061	−.038	−.146*
Role limitations (emotional)	−.161*	.001	.022
Mental health	−.160*	.016	−.085
General health	−.274**	.034	−.058

*$p < .05$; **$p < .01$

Labels: Title, Column headings, Row headings, Footnote, cell, body

Figure 11-1. Parts of table.

The first letter of each major word should be capitalized but not short articles, prepositions, or conjunctions such as "and" and "but."

Body of Table

The body of the table also is referred to as the field (Huth, 1999). The body is the content of the table—its numerical values or words and phrases. The content usually is organized into columns (vertical) and rows (horizontal). The intersection of a column and row, a cell, is where the specific numbers and text are placed. If the cell is empty because the information is not applicable, the cell can be left blank. If the cell is empty because data are missing, however, the author can insert a dash and include a footnote if further explanation is necessary.

Numerical values usually are placed in the columns, which facilitates totaling the scores and percentages. The author should verify that totals and total percentages reflect the numbers and percentages given in the table. When a discrepancy exists, such as the percentages not equaling 100 because of rounding, an explanation can be included in the footnote to the table. Column data should be aligned vertically, for example, by decimal points, so that the numbers are not misinterpreted. This can be seen in the sample tables in this chapter.

Information in the rows of a table should be aligned horizontally to facilitate reading from left to right, across the table. If the lines of text do not fit in the space allotted and run over to the next line, the numbers or words in the cells are placed on the first or top line. For example, in Table 11.2, because the text "Role limitations (physical)" runs over to the next line, the numeric values within the table cells are positioned on the first or top line.

When reporting the results of statistical analyses, the author should consult a style manual or statistics textbook to see what information should be contained in the table. Statistical abbreviations, such as M (mean) and SD (standard deviation), may be used in tables without any explanation in a footnote. A list of statistical abbreviations is provided in Appendix 1.

Other abbreviations, though, may be used in the table but should be described in a footnote, as in the following example of a table footnote:

Note. S = student group; N = registered nurse group.

Column Headings

A table organizes information and presents it logically, and the headings inform the reader about how the information is organized. Each column should have a brief heading that identifies the type of information reported in it. This includes the far left column of the table, referred to as the stub column. For research papers, this column often contains the independent variables. When numerical data are reported in a column, the heading should include the unit of measure, which should be consistent for all of the information in that column. Only one category of information should be reported in a column.

If groups of columns relate to one another, they can be labeled with a heading, and a rule can be placed over the corresponding column headings. For example:

	Education			
Measure	**ADN**	**BSN**	**MSN**	**PhD**

Row Headings

The far left column of a table contains the row headings that describe the content included in the rows of the table. Similar to column headings, these should be brief statements that adequately label the row and all of the items in that row. If groups of rows are related, a heading can be included and subheadings used to clarify this in the table. This can be seen in Table 11.3 where race, highest education, and marital status are used as headings to group the information reported in the rows that follow.

TABLE 11.3

Sample Table With Subheadings to Group Information in Rows

Table 1: Background of Patients Receiving Home Care

Variable	*n*	%
Race		
Caucasian	67	56.8
African American	46	39.0
Hispanic	3	2.5
Asian	2	1.6
Highest education		
<12th grade	40	34.8
High school graduate	64	55.6
College graduate	11	9.6
Marital status		
Married	72	61.0
Divorced/separated	19	16.1
Widowed	9	7.6
Single	18	15.3

Footnotes

Footnotes provide additional details about the table in general or a specific column, row, or entry in the table. They can be used to explain abbreviations in the table, indicate the results of tests of significance, and make the table understandable (Huth, 1999).

Style manuals differ regarding how footnotes are designated. APA's *Publication Manual* (APA, 1994) refers to a footnote pertaining to the entire table as a Note (underlined and followed by a period), which is placed at the bottom of the table. Footnotes for columns, rows, and specific entries are designated by superscript lowercase letters ([a], [b], [c]) placed after the item and then explained at the bottom of the table. The *P* values are designated by asterisks, such as, *$*P < .05$ and **$P < .01$. Sample footnotes are seen in Table 11.4.

Other style manuals use a conventional sequence of footnote symbols. The following symbols are used in the order shown for tables with five or fewer footnotes (AMA, 1998):

* Asterisk

† Dagger

‡ Double dagger

§ Section mark

‖ Parallel mark.

TABLE 11.4

Table With Footnotes

Table 6: Differences in Role Strain Based on Highest Degree of Faculty

Role Strain Scale[a]	BSN		Master's		PhD		F
	M	*SD*	*M*	*SD*	*M*	*SD*	
Role overload	2.89	.69	3.37	.72	3.92	.70	5.96**
Inter-role conflict	2.89	.96	3.46	.89	3.64	.79	3.26*
Inter-sender conflict	2.66	.71	3.13	.78	3.44	.83	3.86**
Total role strain	2.58	.48	2.94	.61	3.12	.43	3.69**

Note. Faculty teaching clinical courses in associate degree and baccalaureate nursing programs.

[a]Developed by Mobily (1991).

*$p < .05$, **$p < .01$

Adapted from: Oermann, M.H. (1998). Role strain of clinical nursing faculty. *Journal of Professional Nursing, 14,* 332. Reprinted by permission of W.B. Saunders.

RELATIONSHIP OF TABLE AND TEXT

Every table must be referred to in the text, and the author should inform readers what to look for in the table. Tables are numbered consecutively, using Arabic numerals, in the order in which they are first mentioned in the text. This number then is used in the text to refer the reader to the table. Two examples follow:

> As seen in Table 1, there were differences between the way men and women perceived the importance of teaching given by the nurse.

> Men and women differed in the importance that they placed on the teaching given by the nurse (Table 3).

When the article is published, tables are placed close to where they are first referenced, as determined by the publisher. Therefore, authors should not write "the table above/below" or the table on "page 7" because it may not be in that place when it is published.

 ## FORMATTING TABLES

Tables are double spaced throughout, including the title and headings. Journals differ in how they format tables, so the author should follow the style manual or use a standard format such as found in this book. Generally, horizontal rules are placed between the table title and column headings to separate the column headings from the body of the table; they also are placed at the bottom of the table to separate it from the footnotes. Rules also are used to group similar columns together, as shown earlier in the chapter. If additional formatting is needed for a particular journal, this will be done by the editor.

Word-processing programs may be used to develop tables, but the author should adhere to the formatting of the style manual. Some word-processing programs enclose tables in boxes, so the author may need to modify this to meet the style requirements. If authors are typing their own manuscripts, they should practice how to develop tables using the word-processing program before beginning to type the manuscript to avoid being distracted during the writing phase.

When submitting the manuscript, each table is placed on a separate page. If tables extend beyond one page, they are continued on the next page and labeled with the table number and title, followed by the word "continued" (Huth, 1999). For wide tables, the author might orient them horizontally (landscape) rather than vertically (portrait), consider preparing two tables, or shift the columns with their headings to the rows, and the rows and headings to the columns if appropriate.

FIGURES

Figures include graphs, charts, diagrams, photographs, maps, and drawings. They can be used to illustrate the findings of a study, display trends in the data, make comparisons, and show equipment, procedures, and other objects described in the text. For research papers, figures allow readers to visualize trends and patterns in the data more easily than a written narrative. An example of a figure is provided in Figure 11-2.

Huth (1999) identified three criteria for deciding whether to use figures in a paper:

- Evidence: Figures should be used only when they present evidence to support conclusions in the paper.
- Efficiency: With some data, figures are more efficient for presenting evidence to support a conclusion than a long discussion in the text, such as when illustrating trends in data over time.

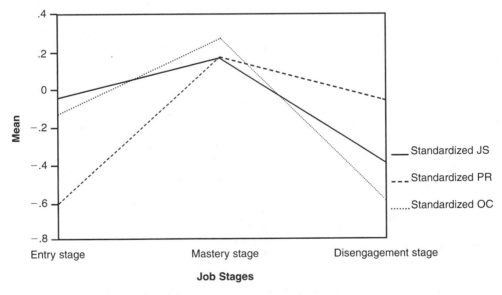

Figure 2. Standardized scores for job satisfaction (JS), productivity (PR), and organizational committment (OC) by job stages.

From McNeese-Smith, D. K., & van Servellen, G. (2000). Age, developmental and job stage influences on nurse outcomes. O*utcomes Management for Nursing Practice, 4*, p. 102. Reprinted by permission of Lippincott Williams & Wilkins.

Figure 11-2. Sample figure.

- Emphasis: Figures can be used to emphasize key points from the paper.

Figures should not be used if the information can be presented as well in the text. Authors should prepare figures only when they are essential to the paper.

Types of Figures

Various types of figures can be prepared, including the following:

- Graphs: Graphs show the relationship of two variables, for example, length of stay in the hospital compared with the number of days on a ventilator. Graphs displaying quantitative data are valuable for indicating changes and patterns in the data. They include line, bar, circle (pie), scatter, and pictorial graphs (APA, 1994).
- Charts: Charts describe the sequence of a process, such as a flowchart to show the steps in a process, and the parts of a structure and their relationships, such as an organizational chart.
- Maps: Maps show relationships and trends that involve locations and distance (AMA, 1998). For instance, they may be used to display the prevalence of health problems in particular communities.
- Drawings: Drawings illustrate an object and its different views. Emphasis can be added and extraneous detail eliminated to make it clear to readers (Pearsall, 1997).
- Photographs: Photographs of patients and objects need to be professionally done and submitted in black and white. Patients must give permission for their photographs to be used in a manuscript.

Guidelines for Developing Figures

How to develop each of the figures described earlier is beyond the scope of this book; this information can be obtained in a style manual. A few general guidelines follow.

- Use large enough letters, numbers, lines, and other symbols so that they can be seen once reduced to fit the journal page. Figures usually are reduced when published, so this should considered when they are constructed. The final printed figures must be easy to read and clear.
- Use standard symbols, such as open and closed circles, triangles, and squares and define them in the legend, or caption, of the figure. Differ-

ent connecting lines also can be used, but Day (1998) cautions authors to use only one set of symbols in a figure.

- If shadings are used, they should be sufficiently different and limited to two or three types in one bar graph. The ideal is to use no shading and black bars (APA, 1994, p. 155).

- Label each axis to indicate what is being measured and the corresponding units.

- Number figures consecutively (eg, Figure 1, Figure 2) and include a title immediately after the number.

- Prepare a legend for each figure, which is placed below the figure. For some illustrations, the legend starts on a separate page (International Committee of Medical Journal Editors [ICMJE], 1997). The figure number, title, and details about the figure are placed in the legend; this is illustrated in Figure 11-2. The legend provides information for understanding the figure and all of the symbols in it without referring to the text.

- Print the figures on bright white paper and submit the originals of all figures with the manuscript. Most figures are reproduced as submitted, so the the original should be without flaws. Figures with the final submission should not be stapled to the manuscript or affixed with paper clips.

- Reformat figures developed for presentations, for example, with Power Point, so the font and layout are consistent with the rest of the paper.

- Paste a label on the back of all figures indicating the number of the figure, author's name, and "top" to show its orientation if relevant (ICMJE, 1997).

- Decide on photographs and special artwork well in advance of submission of the manuscript because of the length of time it takes to receive permission to reprint them or have the artwork prepared (Servodidio, 1998).

 RELATIONSHIP OF FIGURE AND TEXT

Similar to tables, figures are numbered consecutively using Arabic numerals in the order in which they are first mentioned in the text. Every figure is referred to in the text by its number, for example:

> Changes in infant mortality over the time period of the evaluation project are shown in Figure 1.

When the article is published, figures are placed close to where they are first referenced in the text. Similar to tables, authors should not write "the figure above/below" because it may not be in that position when published.

When submitting the manuscript, tables and figures follow the references, with tables first, then figures. Again, tables and figures should be used only when essential, and it is the author's responsibility to know the maximum number allowed in a manuscript.

SUMMARY

Tables are an effective way of presenting detailed and complex information succinctly and clearly. Tables should be used when the author wants to report exact values, present a large amount of detailed information, display different quantitative values simultaneously, and show relationships among data. Tables also are valuable for emphasizing important information from the text. They can be used to highlight key concepts and focus attention on critical points discussed in the paper. Tables should not be used, however, when the information can be better reported in the text.

There are three types of tables: (1) tabulation, a short, informal table developed as part of the text; (2) traditional or formal table, with information arranged in columns and rows; and (3) word or text tables.

Tables contain five major parts: title, body of the table, column headings, row headings, and footnotes. The title should be short, should describe the content in the table, and should be written as a phrase rather than as a sentence. The body or content of the table also is referred to as the field. The content usually is organized into columns (vertical) and rows (horizontal). The intersection of a column and row, a cell, is where the specific numbers and text are placed.

A table provides a way to organize and present information logically, and the headings inform the reader about how the information is organized. Each column has a brief heading that identifies the type of information reported in it. Only one category of information is reported in a column. The far left column of a table contains the row headings that describe the content included in the rows of the table. Footnotes provide additional details about the table in general or about a specific column, row, or entry in the table.

Every table must be referred to in the text, and the author should inform readers what to look for in the table. Tables are numbered consecutively using Arabic numerals in the order in which they are first mentioned in the text. When submitting the manuscript, each table is placed on a separate page after the references.

Figures include graphs, charts, diagrams, photographs, maps, and drawings. They can be used to illustrate the findings of a study, display trends in the data, make comparisons, and show equipment or procedures described in the text.

Figures usually are reduced when published, so the letters, numbers, lines, and symbols should be large enough to be seen easily once reduced to fit the journal page. The legend for the figure is placed below it and includes the figure number, title, and details about the figure. Most figures are reproduced as submitted, so the original should be without flaws. Figures included in the final submission should not be stapled to the manuscript or affixed with paper clips to avoid being damaged.

Similar to tables, figures are numbered consecutively using Arabic numerals in the order in which they are first mentioned in the text. Every figure is referred to in the text by its number. Tables and figures should be used only when essential, and it is the author's responsibility to know the maximum number allowed with a manuscript.

REFERENCES

American Medical Association. (1998). *Manual of style: A guide for authors and editors* (9th ed.). Baltimore: Lippincott Williams & Wilkins.

American Psychological Association (APA). (1994). *Publication manual of the American Psychological Association* (4th ed.). Washington, DC: APA.

Day, R.A. (1998). *How to write and publish a scientific paper* (5th ed.). Phoenix: Oryx Press.

Huth, E.J. (1999). *Writing and publishing in medicine* (3rd ed.). Baltimore: Lippincott Williams & Wilkins.

International Committee of Medical Journal Editors. (1997). Uniform requirements for manuscripts submitted to biomedical journals. *Annals of Internal Medicine, 126*, 36–47. Also available: http://www.icmje.org/

Pearsall, T.E. (1997). *The elements of technical writing.* Boston: Allyn & Bacon.

Servodidio, C.A. (1998). *Writing tips for authors. Insight, 23*(1), 24–27.

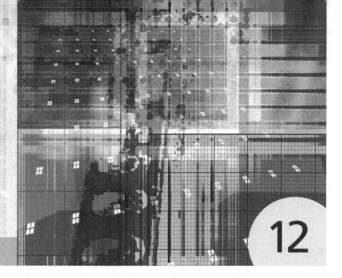

FINAL PAPER AND SUBMISSION TO JOURNAL

12

At this point in the writing process, the author has completed the revisions of the content and format of the paper; has prepared the references, tables, and figures; and is ready to submit the paper to the journal. Before submission, the author has some final responsibilities to ensure that the manuscript is consistent with the journal requirements and contains all required parts. The manuscript then is ready to send to the journal for review.

This chapter describes the steps in preparing the final paper to submit to the journal and the details associated with this submission. A sample cover letter is provided in the chapter, as well as a checklist for authors to ensure that all items are sent with the manuscript, thus avoiding delays in its review.

PREPARATION OF FINAL PAPER

Chapter 9 provides guidelines for revising the content and format of the paper so that it is ready for submission. Because journals differ in their requirements, the author needs to complete a final check of the manuscript to ensure that it is consistent with these requirements. This final check begins by reviewing the guidelines for preparing manuscripts described in the author information page. The author has read this while preparing the manuscript, but the final review confirms that the paper has all essential parts and meets these requirements. The author also notes whether the manuscript may be submitted electronically or in hard copy and how many copies should be sent. Display 12.1 provides a checklist for authors to ensure that the manuscript has the essential parts in the correct order.

> **DISPLAY 12.1** **Order of Parts of Manuscript**
>
> 1. Title page
> 2. Abstract page
> 3. Text
> 4. Acknowledgments
>
> 5. References
> 6. Tables
> 7. Figures

Title Page

Every manuscript needs a title page, which is the first page of the paper. The title page includes the title of the paper; authors' names, credentials, positions, and their affiliated institutions; corresponding author and contact information; and grant or other support. The contact information for the corresponding author must be complete, including name, mailing address, telephone and fax numbers, and email address. For faculty who may not be available during certain times of the year and consultants who are away from the office, home addresses and telephone numbers may be provided to facilitate contact with the editor during these time periods. This also allows for a faster turnaround time for review of page proofs if the manuscript is accepted for publication. If the author received a grant or another type of support for the project reported in the paper, this should be noted on the title page. Display 12.2 provides a sample title page.

The names of the authors and identifying information are included only on the title page, not on the first page of text (Fondiller, 1999). For refereed journals, manuscripts are reviewed anonymously, and the editor removes the title page before sending the paper to the reviewers.

Some journals include a running head, which is a short title placed at the top of each page of the paper (Oermann, 1999). This typically is specified in the information for authors page. When a running head is used, it should be a shorted version of the title because of space limitations (Day, 1998).

Abstract Page

The next page of the paper is the abstract page. How to write the abstract is described earlier in the book. In reviewing the abstract, the author should confirm that the information is consistent with the text. In a sample of 32 manuscripts, Ancker (2000) found that 53% had discrepancies between the abstract and text. The author also should check again that the length of the abstract is within the limits of the journal. Most word-processing programs have a function that allows the author to check the number of words in a document.

DISPLAY 12.2	**Sample Title Page**

Evaluation of Educational Program for Patients with Congestive Heart Failure

Mary Smith, BSN, RN
Clinical Nurse II

John Peterson, MSN, RN, C
Advanced Practice Nurse

Jane Doe, MSN, RN
Nurse Manager

Grace Memorial Hospital
Reading, PA

Correspondence to:
Mary Smith, BSN
[mailing address,
phone and fax numbers,
and email address]

Project supported by Staff Development Department, Grace Memorial Hospital.

The abstract is placed on a separate page after the title page. The heading "Abstract" can be centered at the top of this page. The abstract should be double-spaced, consistent with the rest of the paper.

Text

The next part of the paper is the text. This should be in final form, not requiring further revisions of content, writing style, or format; however, the author should check if headings and subheadings are leveled correctly and if they are typed consistently throughout the manuscript. The author also should check the citations and the consistency between the text and tables and figures.

Headings and Subheadings

Each style manual includes guidelines for determining the level of headings and where to position them in the text. The *Publication Manual of the American Psychological Association* (APA, 1994) describes how to use varied levels of headings in a paper, although for most manuscripts, only two to three levels are needed. The format and placement of the heading depend on its level. For instance, according to the APA, when two levels of heading are used, the first one is centered, and the second-level heading is underlined and placed at the left margin. The text begins on the following line. Third-level headings and beyond are positioned differently in the manuscript.

If using two levels of headings, an alternate way is to position all of the headings and subheadings at the left margin, capitalize the first letter of each word and use lower case letters for the rest, and underline the subheadings so that they are clearly "part" of that section of the text. Another way was proposed by Huth (1999). He recommended typing the headings in all-capital letters, and for subheadings, capitalizing the first letter of each word and using lowercase letters for the rest.

The important point is that headings and subheadings are typed consistently throughout the manuscript, regardless of the format used. It may be helpful to write the headings and subheadings, and their leveling, on a separate sheet of paper to confirm that the content has been organized and divided into sections correctly.

Citations

Although the need for accuracy in preparing citations and references has been discussed throughout the book, the author should check the citations in the text a final time. Citations should be consistent with the style used by the journal, all citations should be included, and they should match the reference on the reference list.

Consistency of Text With Tables and Figures

The need for consistency between the text and related tables and figures has been emphasized in prior chapters. The author should check that the data in the text are consistent with the tables and figures and that each one has been cited accurately in the text. The tables and figures also should be numbered correctly.

Acknowledgments

The next page after the text is acknowledgments, which credits persons who made contributions to the manuscript. These contributions may have come from many areas: consultation on the content of the paper, statistical assistance, editing of the paper, and financial support. Remember that written permission is needed to publish the names of people listed in the acknowledgments.

References

After the acknowledgments is the reference list prepared according to a citation-sequence system, where references are listed in the order in which they are first cited in the text, or according to the name-year system, where they are alphabetized. The author already should have verified the accuracy of the references against the original documents, but if this was not done previously, it is an important step in preparing the final copy for submission. The author also checks that each reference on the list is cited at the correct place in the text, the reference format is consistent with the journal requirements and style manual, and each reference includes complete information.

Manuscripts cited in the text that still are in the process of being published can be included on the reference list with "in press" inserted at the end of the reference. Style manuals provide formats for listing papers under review and unpublished works in the reference section.

Tables

Each table is typed on a separate page and numbered consecutively in the order in which they appear in the text. The author checks that the tables are cited in the text at the correct place and that the information in the table supports the text. The author also should review the titles of the tables and check that they are formatted consistently with the style used by the journal or according to the general principles provided here. The author should have identified earlier how many tables and figures are allowed with each manuscript, but if this has not been done, this limit should be confirmed before submitting the manuscript.

Figures

Figures follow the tables when submitting the manuscript, with each figure placed on a separate page similar to the tables. Figures are numbered consecutively in the order in which they are cited in the text. Remember not to staple or use paper clips to affix the original figures to the manuscript because the figures might become damaged.

TYPING FINAL MANUSCRIPT

The manuscript must be typed according to the journal specifications in the information for authors page. Papers are double-spaced throughout, beginning with the title page and continuing through the last page of the manuscript. This includes double-spacing the references, tables, and figure captions. Double-spacing is used for the references themselves, not only to separate each reference on the list.

Authors should consider other important guidelines for keyboarding the paper. If the paper is too long, do not include more lines per page by using narrow margins. The journal guidelines may specify the size of the margins, but if unsure, refer to the style manual or use 1- to 1½-inch margins on all sides.

Paragraphs should be indented, and spaces should not be left between each paragraph. Words should not be divided at the end of a line; most word-processing programs take care of this. Pages should be left-justified (aligning the text at the left margin), not right-justified. When right-justified, there may be large spaces between words and symbols in a line.

Pages are numbered consecutively, considering the title page as the first page. Some journals specify the placement of page numbers, but if not indicated in the author guidelines, pages can be numbered in the right-hand corner of each page, either at the top or bottom.

The hard copies of the manuscript should be printed on a high-quality white paper. A laser or ink-jet printer should be used (Huth, 1999). Dot-matrix printers are acceptable only if they are letter quality. After printing the necessary number of copies, the author should check each page of each copy to be sure that it has printed correctly and pages are in the correct order. Some authors prefer to print an original and make copies to submit with it. This same principle holds true: each page of each copy should be checked as well as their order. Co-authors should have a final copy of the paper for their files.

Some journals allow electronic submission of manuscripts; others may request both a hard copy of the paper and one on a floppy disk. This information is indicated in the author guidelines.

The author should not place the completed paper in a cover or binder (McConnell, 1999). Except for the originals of the figures, the paper may be stapled or paper clipped.

 ## SUBMISSION OF MANUSCRIPT TO JOURNAL

The paper now is ready to send to the journal. Submission to the journal requires writing a cover letter to accompany the manuscript, obtaining signatures on the transfer of copyright form if required for submission, packing the manuscript and related materials, and mailing it. These steps are described in this section of the chapter.

Cover Letter

The cover letter accompanies the manuscript and provides the editor with information about the paper and corresponding author (Display 12.3). The cover letter should include the following:

- Title of the paper
- Department of the journal to which it has been submitted for consideration, if relevant
- A statement that paper is original and has not been published already

---

DISPLAY 12.3	**Sample Cover Letter**

March 14, 2002

Dr. Marilyn Oermann
Editor, *Outcomes Management*
5557 Cass
Detroit, MI 48202

Dear Dr. Oermann:

Enclosed please find four copies of the manuscript, "Evaluation of Educational Program for Patients with Congestive Heart Failure," for your review for possible publication in *Outcomes Management*. Neither the entire paper nor any part of its content has been published or has been accepted by another journal. The manuscript is submitted only to this journal.

Thank you for your consideration.

Sincerely,

Mary Smith
1221 Cranbrook Road
Reading, PA 19709
313.677.4309

John Peterson
John Peterson

Jane Doe
Jane Doe

- Corresponding author's full name, affiliation, and complete contact information
- The number of copies and other materials submitted.

The cover letter does not need to be long but should contain the information just listed. The complete title of the paper should be specified in the letter. If the title does not explain fully all of the content in the manuscript or how the paper might be acceptable to a department of the journal, the author might include a few sentences describing the focus of the paper. In the sample letter in Display 12.3, the article title "Evaluation of Educational Program for Patients With Congestive Heart Failure" may not sufficiently explain that the program begins during the patient's hospitalization, continues through home care, and includes periodic teaching and follow-up using telephone contact with the patient. A sentence to this effect might be included in the cover letter.

Some journals have departments that publish different types of articles. For example, *Applied Nursing Research* (ANR) accepts papers in three main categories: original research, clinical methods, and research briefs (ANR, 2000). The *Journal of Obstetric, Gynecologic, and Neonatal Nursing* (JOGNN) has several areas for submissions: Principles and Practices, Clinical Studies, Thoughts and Opinions, Case Reports, and In Review (integrated literature reviews) (JOGNN, 2000). The cover letter should indicate if the paper was written for a particular department.

Because of issues with duplicate publications, discussed in the beginning of this book, authors should include a statement in the cover letter indicating that the paper is original and has not been published already in its entirety or in part. A sample statement is, "Neither the entire paper nor any part of its content has been published or has been accepted by another journal. The manuscript is submitted only to this journal." The sample cover letter in Display 12.3 includes this statement.

Some journals also may require a statement in the cover letter indicating any publications that are based on the same data set or have similar content. In this case, the author should indicate exactly how the manuscript differs from these other publications. Journals also may ask the author to submit these articles with the manuscript.

The cover letter also should specify the full name and affiliation of the corresponding author. Contact information, including mailing address, telephone and fax numbers, and email address, should be included; this information should be consistent with that listed on the title page. A home address and number may be provided or an alternate individual may be listed for contact if the corresponding author is unavailable.

For papers written by more than one author, the uniform requirements specify that the cover letter be signed by each author (International Committee of Medical Journal Editors, 1997). A clear designation of the corresponding author is important so that the editor knows who to contact.

The cover letter also includes the number of copies of the manuscript and other materials submitted with the manuscript.

Financial Disclosure

If there were any financial or contractual associations between the authors and others that might bias the study or interpretations of findings, they should be disclosed to the editor (Huth, 1999). A statement may be included in the cover letter, and the authors may be asked to sign a separate form to this effect. For example, the guidelines for *AORN Journal* (AORN, 2000) direct the author to disclose if there was a financial association between the author and the commercial company that makes the product featured in the manuscript.

In addition to financial interest, authors need to disclose any other type of involvement that might represent a potential conflict of interest, such as being a paid consultant on a project evaluated highly in the manuscript, owning stock in the company that manufactures the product described in the paper, or receiving an honorarium for participating in the evaluation of the product. For example, a statement such as this might be included in the cover letter:

> Ms. Smith is a consultant for Software Incorporated, which produces the software evaluated in this paper.

The author also might include a statement in the cover letter indicating that there is no commercial, proprietary, or financial interest in the product or subject matter discussed in the paper (American Medical Association, 1998).

Copyright

For some journals, the author submits the signed transfer of copyright form with the submission, whereas for others this is completed only when the paper is accepted for publication. If the copyright form is needed for submission, this will be noted on the author guidelines and probably will be available at the journal's Web site. If not, the author needs to obtain the copyright transfer form from the editorial office. This should have been done when the journal was selected so that it is available when the manuscript is ready to be sent.

Materials to Send

With the cover letter completed, the author is ready to prepare the other materials to submit. The author must send the correct number of copies of the paper as specified in the author guidelines; remember to check each copy to ensure that it has all of the pages in the correct order.

If the manuscript includes original figures, they can be placed in a separate, clearly labeled envelope. Copies of the figures may be included with each copy of the manuscript as long as the editor has the original illustrations. Be careful when packaging the manuscript to protect the originals from damage during mailing. Cardboard can be placed in the envelope to avoid bending them.

Other materials submitted are the permissions to reprint information in the manuscript, letters granting permission to publish the acknowledgments and to cite the names of institutions in the manuscript, and permissions to publish photographs and other illustrations. If requested by the journal, the author should include the transfer of copyright form.

If the journal requires hard copies of the manuscript and a copy on a floppy disk, the disk should be labeled clearly with the author's name, title of the manuscript, platform (PC or MAC), and software program (eg, Microsoft Word or Word Perfect, including the version number). A new disk should be used, and it should be packaged in a mailing folder to avoid damage. For other journals, submissions may be done electronically, although some of the materials such as permission letters need to be mailed.

Although many editors acknowledge receipt of the manuscript electronically, some do not, and some authors may not have email addresses. If unsure how the editor handles this, the author should insert a reply postcard or self-addressed, stamped envelope.

Manuscripts are not returned if rejected. If the author wants the original of the paper returned, a self-addressed and stamped envelope should be sent with the submission package. Display 12.4 provides a checklist for authors to use to confirm that they are sending the required materials.

Mailing Package

For the first submission, when there is no deadline, the materials can be mailed first class. Subsequently, when there are deadlines, express mail might be worth the additional cost. Authors should have one complete copy of all materials mailed, not only the manuscript itself.

 ## SUMMARY

The author needs to complete a final check of the manuscript to ensure that it is consistent with the requirements of the journal specified in the information for authors page. This final review confirms that the paper has all essential parts and meets these requirements. The author also notes whether the manuscript may be submitted electronically or in hard copy only and how many copies are sent.

DISPLAY 12.4 **Checklist for Submission of Materials**

✔ Cover letter
✔ Correct number of copies of manuscript
✔ Original figures in separate envelope labeled clearly
✔ Permissions letters
✔ Transfer of copyright form (if requested at time of submission)
✔ Floppy disk version of manuscript (if requested)
✔ Reply postcard or self-addressed, stamped envelope (to acknowledge receipt of manuscript)
✔ Self-addressed, stamped envelope for return of the original manuscript after the review (if desired)

The author should check the title page, abstract page, and text. Although the manuscript should be in final form, not requiring any further revisions of content, writing style, or format, the author should check the following: (1) leveling of the headings and subheadings—they should be typed consistently throughout the manuscript, (2) citations, and (3) consistency between the text and any tables and figures.

The next page after the text is acknowledgments, which credits persons who made contributions to the manuscript. Written permissions are needed for these acknowledgments.

After the acknowledgments is the reference list, which is prepared according to a citation-sequence system, where references are listed in the order in which they are first cited in the text, or name-year system, where they are alphabetized. The author should complete one last check that the references are accurate, each reference on the list is cited at the correct place in the text, the reference format is consistent with the journal requirements and style used for preparation, and each reference is complete.

Each table and figure is submitted on a separate page and numbered consecutively in the order in which it appears in the text. The author checks that the tables and figures are numbered consistently with their placement in the text.

The manuscript should be typed according to the journal specifications. Papers are double-spaced throughout, beginning with the title page and continuing through the last page of the manuscript. This includes double-spacing the references, tables, and figure captions. Margins should be between 1 and 1½ inches wide on all sides. Pages should be left-justified (aligning the text at the left margin) and numbered consecutively, beginning with the title page.

Journals differ in the format allowed for papers to be submitted; some require hard copies only, others ask for hard copies and a copy on a floppy disk, and still others provide an opportunity to submit electronically. The hard copies of the manuscript should be printed on a high-quality white paper. After printing the necessary number of copies, the author should check each page of each copy to be sure that it has printed correctly and pages are in the correct order. Authors should print copies for their files and those of the co-authors.

Submission to the journal requires writing a cover letter to accompany the manuscript, obtaining signatures on the transfer of copyright form if required for submission, packing the manuscript and related materials, and mailing it. The author now awaits the results of the review of the paper.

REFERENCES

American Medical Association. (1998). *Manual of style: A guide for authors and editors* (9th ed.). Baltimore: Lippincott Williams & Wilkins.

American Psychological Association (APA). (1994). *Publication manual of the American Psychological Association* (4th ed.). Washington, DC: APA.

Ancker, J. (2000). Frequency of selected arithmetic and reporting problems in medical manuscripts: A descriptive study. *American Medical Writers Association Journal, 15*(3), 24–27.

Author guidelines. (2000). AORN online. [On-line]. Available: *http://www.aorn.org/journal/guidelines.htm*. Accessed March 17, 2000.

Author guidelines. (2000). Applied Nursing Research. [On-line]. Available: *http://www.appliednursingresearch.org*. Accessed October 2, 2000.

Author guidelines. (2000). Journal of Obstetric, Gynecologic, and Neonatal Nursing (JOGNN). [On-line]. Available: *http://www.nursingcenter.com/journals/author.cfm*. Accessed September 29, 2000.

Day, R.A. (1998). *How to write and publish a scientific paper* (5th ed.). Phoenix, AZ: Oryx Press.

Fondiller, S.H. (1999). *The writer's workbook* (2nd ed.). Sudbury, MA: Jones & Bartlett.

Huth, E.J. (1999). *Writing and publishing in medicine* (3rd ed.). Baltimore: Lippincott Williams & Wilkins.

International Committee of Medical Journal Editors. (1997). Uniform requirements for manuscripts submitted to biomedical journals. *Annals of Internal Medicine, 126*, 36–47. Also available: http://www.icmje.org/

McConnell, C.R. (1999). From idea to print: Writing for a professional journal. *Health Care Supervisor, 17*(3), 72–85.

Oermann, M.H. (1999). Writing for publication as an advanced practice nurse. *Nursing Connections, 12*(3), 5–13.

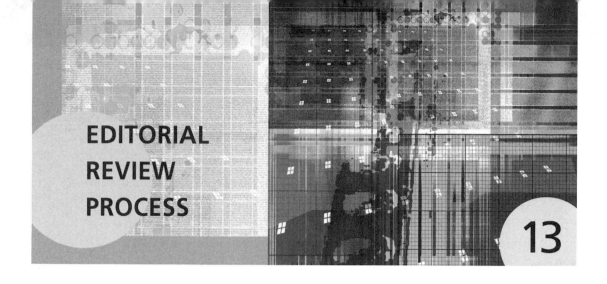

EDITORIAL REVIEW PROCESS

13

Chapter 12 presented the final steps in preparing a paper for submission to a journal. This same process is used in writing other types of papers such as a grant or a report for an organization. When the paper is completed, another person or group is likely to read and critique it, whether for publication, funding, or another purpose. The process of writing drafts and revising them for content and format has been emphasized in earlier chapters, so that the final paper contains the essential content, is organized clearly, and is well written. The cycle of writing a draft and revising it, combined with attention to other details described earlier, results in a paper that should be competitive with others.

This chapter presents the editorial review process from the point at which the paper is received in the journal office through the final editorial decision. The roles and responsibilities of the editor, editorial board, and peer reviewers are discussed, and examples are provided of criteria used by reviewers when asked to critique a manuscript for publication. The peer review process is not without issues, which are examined in the chapter.

Manuscripts submitted to a journal may be accepted without revision or accepted provisionally pending revision, may be returned to the author for a major revision and resubmission, or may be rejected. Each of these editorial decisions has implications for the author and the author's response to the editor.

WHO IS INVOLVED?

When the manuscript is completed and all materials are assembled, the manuscript package is sent to the editor of the journal to begin the review process.

The manuscript arrives at the editorial office, which might include a large staff for journals widely circulated and published frequently, or at an office with an editor and limited support staff. Journals differ in the resources needed to process manuscripts and prepare them for production once accepted. For example, health-related newspapers and journals published monthly need more editorial staff to handle the number of manuscripts to be processed compared with a specialty nursing journal published quarterly. The number of people involved in the editorial process and their roles, therefore, differ based on the needs of the journal.

Editor

The editor of a nursing journal is an expert in the nursing specialty or content area covered by the journal. Depending on the focus of the journal, editors may have expertise in clinical practice, administration, management, education, or research. Few nursing editors have trained specifically to become editors; most are selected for the position because of their knowledge of the topics covered by the journal.

In addition to content expertise, editors usually have additional knowledge and skills related to the types of articles published in the journal. For example, editors of journals that publish research have an understanding of statistics and research methods and may have conducted research themselves. Clinical journals that focus on a particular nursing role, such as publications for nurse practitioners, generally are edited by someone functioning in that role or with an understanding of it.

To maintain their expertise, editors spend much of their time keeping current by reading the professional literature; by attending professional meetings; through their own research, writing, and work; and by maintaining contact with experts in the field. This also enables them to solicit manuscripts for the journal.

Some editors of journals began initially as assistant or associate editors, then moved into the editor's position. Most, however, served on editorial or advisory boards of journals, were manuscript reviewers, and have experience themselves writing publications such as articles or books.

Blancett (1997) referred to editors as gatekeepers of nursing knowledge because they decide which papers are to be published and, therefore, what people will be reading about a topic (p. 16). In this sense, editors contribute to the development of nursing knowledge and to changes in practice, administration, and teaching.

Functions of Editors

Some editors work full time as editors, although most function as part-time editors who hold other positions in nursing (Fondiller, 1999). Part-time editors are given an honorarium by the publisher for serving in that role. The publisher of the journal is the individual or group that produces, distributes, and markets the journal. Editors report to the publisher of the journal through different types of organizational arrangements.

The editor is accountable to the readers for quality manuscripts that promote the development of the field. The editor also is accountable to the editorial board and reviewers for carrying out the editorial process and arriving at decisions consistent with their recommendations and advice. Because editors report to the publisher, they are responsible for meeting the publisher's expectations associated with editing the journal.

Responsibilities of the Editor

The primary responsibilities of the editor are to

- Solicit manuscripts
- Work with authors to develop their ideas into manuscripts that are suitable for publication
- Assess the quality of manuscripts submitted to the journal
- Select reviewers to critique papers
- Decide on manuscripts to publish based on recommendations from the reviewers
- Edit manuscripts
- Decide on the papers to include in each issue
- Complete other tasks to prepare the manuscripts for publication.

Blancett (1997) emphasized that the editor assumes overall responsibility for the editorial content and quality of the journal.

With most journals, the editor is responsible for deciding whether to accept or reject a manuscript. With refereed journals, peer reviewers critique the submitted manuscript and advise the editor on the acceptance decision, but the editor makes the final decision. For tenure and promotion considerations, refereed publications carry more weight because they include this peer review process, thereby providing an external review of the quality of the work and its contribution to nursing. Other journals, though, are not peer reviewed, and the editors read and critique the manuscripts in-house and make the acceptance decisions. These are considered nonrefereed journals.

Editors work with authors, editorial board members, peer reviewers, and the production editor. Because the editor interfaces with the production editor, there is an opportunity to maintain the quality of the content of the manuscript as it moves through production.

The editor also establishes the editorial policies for the journal and develops the author guidelines for submitting manuscripts. These policies and guidelines generally are prepared with input from the editorial board and peer reviewers. If the journal is an official publication of a professional organization, the editor works closely with the officers and board of the organization so that consistency is maintained between the goals of the journal and those of the organization.

In some journals, the editor writes an editorial or solicits other people to write it. When associated with a nursing organization, the editorials often reflect the positions of that organization.

For journals with columns and departments, the editor has a role in soliciting manuscripts for them or in working with the assistant or associate editor who has this responsibility. The editor and assistant or associate editor review these papers and suggest revisions to the authors rather than sending them to peer reviewers for critique.

Managing Editor

In addition to the editor, some journals also have a managing editor who is a paid professional responsible for the administrative details associated with processing the manuscripts from submission through publication. The managing editor sends the manuscripts to reviewers, tracks the status of reviews, and oversees the processing of the manuscripts once accepted for publication. Through the work of the managing editor, the manuscript is converted from an accepted paper to a published one (Day, 1998).

Editorial Board

Editors do not make decisions in isolation about the journals they edit. They consult with an editorial board, whose members have expertise on the content covered by the journal, as well as the expertise needed for reviewing the quality, accuracy, and timeliness of manuscripts submitted to the journal. The editor makes the decisions as to who will serve on the editorial or advisory board to the journal.

The editorial board gives the editor advice on general policies concerning the journal (Barnum, 1995). This advice may include suggestions on the future directions of the journal, types of articles to be published, focus of columns and departments, and guidelines and criteria for manuscript review.

PEER REVIEW

The International Committee of Medical Journal Editors [ICMJE] (1997) defined peer review journals as ones in which most of the published articles are reviewed by experts who are not part of the editorial staff. The process by which these journals review manuscripts, and their related policies, differ widely across journals. Therefore, general principles of peer review are described, recognizing that each journal has its own way of conducting peer reviews, its own criteria, and its own format. Some journals publish statements in the information for authors page on their peer review process and policies.

Peer review began in the 18th century when committees were set up by medical societies to evaluate papers sent to them for publication in their journals (Kronick, 1990). As medicine became more specialized and more journals developed, editors found that they lacked the knowledge to review manuscripts out of their specialization and sought experts to give them opinions about the submitted papers. Specialization became a driving force in the acceptance of peer review (Manske, 1997). As more manuscripts became available, peer review also was seen as a way of accepting the best papers for the journal.

Blind Review Process

Many peer reviewed journals use a process of blind review in which submitted manuscripts are sent to reviewers with the identity of the author and institution concealed. The editor removes the title page and conceals other identifying information. The principle behind sending a "blinded" copy, free of identifying information, is that there is less chance of bias when the reviewer does not know who wrote the article or the author's credentials.

Blinding of authorship does not always work because in specialized areas, the reviewers often know the research and projects of others (Baggs, 1999). Yankauer (1991) reported that reviewers frequently could identify the authors even when a blinded copy was sent. Most reviewers could identify who wrote the paper from the self-referencing (62%). Even so, blind review was favored by 75% of the reviewers in the study because they believed it eliminated bias. Reasons for opposing blind review was that blinding was not possible, and identification of the author either did not affect judgment or assisted reviewers in evaluating a paper.

Reviewers also are unknown to the author. When reviews are returned to the author, the identities of the reviewers are masked so that the author does not know who read the paper. With this anonymity, reviewers are free to evaluate a paper honestly and without fear of repercussions from the author if they give a negative review. These reviews are believed to be fairer. Thomas (1998) emphasized that without an anonymous review, there may be greater hesitancy to make critical comments to an author, particularly if the reviewer and author know each other professionally.

Unfortunately, some authors have received highly critical reviews but without the feedback needed to improve the manuscript. Blackwell (2000) questioned if the process of disguising reviewers' identities—intended to encourage giving their opinions honestly—may have created a system in which some reviewers are too critical.

Reviewers are chosen by the editor because of their expertise to critique the manuscript. In one study, 102 manuscripts were reviewed blind by referees selected by journal editors and referees chosen by the paper's principal author (Earnshaw et al., 2000). Manuscripts were read using a standard review form; rated on originality, clinical importance, and clarity; and given a final overall recommendation about possible publication. Reviewers chosen by the editor were more critical of the submitted manuscripts than those selected by the authors themselves. The researchers concluded that the constructive criticism given by reviewers whose identities are unknown to the author is of value in improving the final paper and assisting the editor in making the acceptance decision.

Some believe that concealing the identities of authors and masking reviewers' identities improve the quality of the review, but van Rooyen, Godlee, Evans, Smith, and Black (1998) did not find this to be true. They conducted a study of 527 manuscripts randomly allocated to three groups: unmasked (revealing the identity of the reviewer to a co-reviewer), masked (concealing the reviewer's identity), or uninformed that a study was taking place. Two reviewers for each manuscript were randomly assigned to read either a blinded or unblinded version of the paper. There were no differences in the quality of the reviews between blinded and unblinded or between masked and unmasked groups. Justice et al. (1998) also found that concealing the identity of the author to reviewers did not produce higher quality reviews.

Whether there was less bias, though, was not studied. In Yankauer's (1991) research, respondents supported blind review because they believed that it eliminated bias. Research on the effects of blind review on bias and quality needs to be conducted in nursing and other fields.

Purposes of Peer Review

The review process assists the editor in establishing the importance of the paper, its relevance to the journal, value of its content to readers, timeliness of the manuscript, and overall quality, thereby providing a basis for the acceptance decision. Peer reviewers give the editor and author their judgment and expert opinions about the manuscript. The editor uses the review as a basis for making the acceptance decision, and authors use the review for revising the paper.

With some journals, reviewers do not state their judgments on whether the paper should be published. For others, reviewers recommend to the editor if the manuscript should be accepted, revised, or rejected; the editor then makes the acceptance decision considering these recommendations. Even though reviewers give advice to the editor, they usually do not "vote" on whether to accept a manuscript (Huth, 1999). Editors are more likely to publish papers when both reviewers recommend acceptance than when they disagree or recommend rejection (Rothwell & Martyn, 2000).

Journals differ in the focus of the manuscript reviews according to the types of articles that they publish. Journals that publish clinical articles emphasize the practical implications of the paper and how the ideas might be used by readers. Reviewers for journals that publish research focus more on the adequacy of the research design, how the research was carried out, appropriateness of the statistical methods, and conclusions drawn from the evidence.

Although there are differences across journals, reviewers commonly evaluate if the

- Ideas and information in the paper are new and innovative
- Paper contributes to the nursing field and to readers' knowledge and skills
- Content is important and warrants publication
- Content is relevant to the journal's readers
- Content is at the appropriate level for readers
- Content is applicable for the reader's practice
- Paper is well organized
- Ideas are expressed clearly and developed logically
- Research methods are adequate
- Evidence is sufficient to support conclusions drawn from the research
- References are current (within the last 5 years) and relevant.

Peer Reviewers

Rarely does the editor possess the expertise to critique the different types of manuscripts and range of topics submitted to the journal. Therefore, journals rely on external or peer reviewers, sometimes called referees, to read and critically judge the manuscripts submitted to the journal.

Peer reviewers are experts in the topic of the manuscript; they are considered "peers" of the author because they have similar expertise allowing them to critique the paper. Depending on the journal and type of manuscript, peer reviewers may have published on the topic, may be practicing in the same specialization as the focus of the manuscript, or may have research or statistical expertise needed for the review. The principle is that peer reviewers have expertise to critique the manuscript and make recommendations to the editor.

The panel of peer reviewers of a journal usually is larger than the editorial board because expertise is needed for a wide range of topics. The editor also may ask ad hoc reviewers, people who do not serve on the review panel but have specialized areas of expertise, to read a particular manuscript. With some journals, the editorial board also serves as the review panel, with the board members reviewing manuscripts in their areas of specialization.

Peer reviewers are chosen by the editor based on their expertise. Persons may be suggested to serve as peer reviewers by the assistant and associate editors of the journal, editorial board members, and current manuscript reviewers. Often, reviewers have written for the journal and therefore are known by the editor for their particular expertise.

Review Forms and Guidelines

Most journals use review forms that specify the criteria for judging the manuscript and provide space for reviewers to support their ratings with comments about the paper. Examples of forms from different types of journals are in shown in Figure 13-1. These review forms and narrative comments are returned to the author for use in revising the paper. They also provide documentation for the editorial decision. With some journals, reviewers write their comments directly on the manuscript pages, which also are returned to the author for feedback.

Peer reviewers follow exact guidelines to ensure that reviews are fair and unbiased. Reviews are done consistently for each manuscript submitted using the same process, criteria, and format. Reviewers disclose to the editor any conflict of interest that would bias their judgment of the manuscript and disqualify themselves from the review process (ICMJE, 1997).

Editors, editorial board members, and peer reviewers treat manuscripts and reviews as privileged communication. The manuscript is not publicly discussed before publication, and reviewers are not allowed to copy the submitted manuscript, use the ideas in their own work, or share the ideas with others (ICMJE, 1997).

 MANUSCRIPT REVIEW PROCESS

When the manuscript arrives in the editorial office of the journal, it is given a number, which is used throughout the review process to track the manuscript. This number is recorded on the letter to the author acknowledging receipt of the manuscript and should be used by the author in subsequent correspondence with the editor.

Authors should receive a letter acknowledging receipt of the manuscript within a few weeks after sending it. After this time, the author should contact the editorial office to confirm that the manuscript package arrived and is being processed. The author should note the manuscript number and should keep all correspondence regarding the manuscript.

(text continues on page 260)

NURSE EDUCATOR *MANUSCRIPT REVIEW FORM*

*Reviewer*_____ *Date* _____

Title _____

As you read, write positive, negative, and developmental comments on the manuscript pages. Return manuscript pages with comments; destroy remaining pages of manuscript.

Yes	No	
____	____	Does the paper present new findings or ideas?
____	____	If no, does it present old material better?
		Is the content:
____	____	timely/relevant?
____	____	logically and clearly developed?
____	____	sophisticated enough for our readers?
____	____	innovative?
____	____	on cutting edge of knowledge on topic?
____	____	Introduction—is the purpose of the paper clear?
____	____	Methods (if applicable)
____	____	Are the sample and sampling method adequate?
____	____	Are the instruments reliable and valid?
____	____	Are statistical tests appropriate?
____	____	Do conclusions/generalizations/implications go beyond what findings/data/theory support?
____	____	Are most references from the last 3 years?
____	____	Are the references relevant?
____	____	Is the content's application/utility made explicit to the reader's practice setting?
____	____	If there is no cost-benefit analysis, does the content warrant its addition?
____	____	Was the paper interesting to read?

Recommendation:
( ) Must publish ___ with ___ without revisions (innovative, seminal paper)
( ) Publish after satisfactory revision (but topic/approach in literature)
( ) Review again after major revision
( ) Reject

Please circle the number that best indicates the overall quality of this manuscript:

1	2	3	4	5	6
Outstanding	Excellent	Good	Acceptable	Uncertain of acceptability	Unacceptable

Comments/Suggestions:

Figure 13-1 (A). Sample manuscript review form. Form A developed by Suzanne Smith, Editor-in-Chief, *Nurse Educator* and *Journal of Nursing Administration.* Reprinted by permission of S. Smith and Lippincott Williams & Wilkins.

NURSING RESEARCH *REVIEW FORM*
1ST REVIEW

Manuscript #

Manuscript title:

Reviewer:

Please evaluate the following by placing an X in the correct box:

	Adequate	Inadequate (please describe in written review)	Not appropriate (please describe in written review)
Problem statement			
Attention to relevant literature			
Theoretical framework			
Research design			
Data analysis			
Organization			
Writing style			

	lowest 1	2	3	4	highest 5
Value of topic					
Probable reader interest in topic					
Importance of present contribution to nursing					
Priority of topic for publication					
Rank this manuscript for its value					

Reviewer's Recommendation (please place an X in the appropriate box):

☐ Accept without revisions   ☐ Maybe accept with revisions

☐ Accept with revisions   ☐ Do not accept

Please provide a comprehensive and integrated review of this manuscript.
Be sure to present a balanced view of the manuscript's strengths and w   .

Figure 13-1 (B). Sample manuscript review form. Form B reprinted by permission of M.C. Dougherty, Editor of *Nursing Research*, and Lippincott Williams & Wilkins.

Manuscript No. _____

Clinical Nurse Specialist *Manuscript Evaluation Form*

These pages are to record your evaluation of the manuscript and to provide your comments to the Associate Editor and the Editors. This document will be returned to the author(s) of the manuscript. Written comments are extremely helpful to provide the author(s) with constructive feedback. Rate the manuscript on the following items using the Likert scale as indicated below by circling the appropriate number. Additional written comments may be made in the space provided.

Structure/Style

1. The construction, including introduction, body of the paper, and conclusion, is:

		Insufficient		Adequate		Excellent	Written comments
a	Organized	1	2	3	4	5	
b.	Logically developed	1	2	3	4	5	
c.	Complete	1	2	3	4	5	
d.	Concise	1	2	3	4	5	
e.	Clear	1	2	3	4	5	
f.	Grammatically correct	1	2	3	4	5	

2. The title and the abstract are:

a.	Informative	1	2	3	4	5
b.	Concise	1	2	3	4	5
c.	Clear	1	2	3	4	5
d.	Complete	1	2	3	4	5
e.	Representative of content	1	2	3	4	5

3. The text, tables, or illustrations are:

a.	Easy to follow	1	2	3	4	5
b.	Clearly designed	1	2	3	4	5
c.	Relevant	1	2	3	4	5
d.	Adequately captioned	1	2	3	4	5
e.	Too few	1	2	3	4	5
f.	Too many	1	2	3	4	5

Figure 13-1 (C). Sample manuscript review form. Form C developed by Pauline C. Beecroft. Reprinted by permission of Pauline C. Beecroft, Editor, *Clinical Nurse Specialist*, and by Lippincott Williams & Wilkins.

Content

1. The idea, issue, or topic is:

	Poor		Adequate		Excellent	Written comments
a. Original	1	2	3	4	5	
b. Important	1	2	3	4	5	
c. Relevant to CNS practice	1	2	3	4	5	
d. Timely	1	2	3	4	5	

2. When compared to similar literature, is the theoretical foundation of the content:

a. Scientifically based	1	2	3	4	5
b. Adequately referenced	1	2	3	4	5
c. Congruent with similar literature	1	2	3	4	5
d. Interpreted correctly	1	2	3	4	5
e. Free from technical errors	1	2	3	4	5

Overall evaluation of the manuscript:

Figure 13-1 (C) *Continued.*

Careful records are established by the editor or managing editor so that each copy of the manuscript can be tracked through the review process beginning with its arrival at the editorial office, through the review and revision stages, and into production. For larger journals, the managing editor usually assumes this responsibility. This record system is followed carefully so that the whereabouts of each copy of the manuscript is known at all times, and devices are built into the system to signal delays in reviews (Day, 1998).

Reasons Manuscripts Returned to Author

Not all manuscripts are sent out for review. If the manuscript is not relevant for the journal, the editor is likely to return it to the author without its being reviewed. In the letter to the author, the editor usually specifies why the manuscript is not suitable for the journal and its readers. The author, however, can avoid this situation by carefully selecting journals for submission, as discussed earlier in the book.

The second reason that a manuscript may be returned to the author is when it is incomplete or does not conform to the journal requirements. Perhaps too few copies were submitted, pages may have been missing, or the reference format may not have been consistent with the journal guidelines. The importance of carefully preparing the manuscript and checking it before sub-

Cancer Nursing: *An International Journal for Cancer Care*

Summary Review

Please rate the quality of this manuscript on the following factors:

	High				Low
1. Significance of topic	5	4	3	2	1
2. Appropriateness of CANCER NURSING	5	4	3	2	1
3. Author's demonstration of authority	5	4	3	2	1
4. Clarity/writing style	5	4	3	2	1
5. Organization of material	5	4	3	2	1
6. Usefulness for practitioners	5	4	3	2	1
7. (For research reports only)	5	4	3	2	1
a. clarity of objectives	5	4	3	2	1
b. conceptual/theoretical framework	5	4	3	2	1
c. operationalization of variables	5	4	3	2	1
d. sample/sample selection	5	4	3	2	1
e. methodology	5	4	3	2	1
f. data analysis	5	4	3	2	1
g. conclusions/implications	5	4	3	2	1
8. Overall priority for publication	5	4	3	2	1

Reviewer's signature:_____   Date returned:_____

Please annotate the manuscript with your questions and/or comments. Detailed comments and suggestions for improvement of the manuscript should be written out below and/or on the back of this form.

Figure 13-1 (D). Sample manuscript review form. Form D reprinted by permission of Carol Reed Ash, Editor of *Cancer Nursing*, and Lippincott Williams & Wilkins.

mission is described earlier. If authors do not follow these principles, the review of the manuscript may be delayed.

Steps in Review Process

After the editor determines the suitability of the manuscript for the journal, the review process begins. The number of peer reviews performed depends on the journal, but generally at least two reviews of each manuscript are completed.

For some papers, an additional review might be included to assess a specific aspect of the paper, such as the statistical analysis used for a research study.

The editor decides who should review the manuscript. This decision is based on who has the expertise to evaluate the manuscript and make a judgment of its relevance for readers, importance, timeliness, and quality. For papers with highly specialized content, the editor may seek ad hoc reviewers, people not on the review panel who normally do not review for the journal. They may have the expertise, however, to judge a particular manuscript.

The results of the peer review then are sent to the author with the editorial decision on whether the paper is accepted, should be revised and resubmitted, or is rejected. The editor also sends questions about the content, issues to be resolved, and suggestions for revision that were identified during the review process. The reviews provide data for the editor to use in making an acceptance decision and feedback for authors in revising the paper to strengthen it. In some instances, the manuscript may be accepted without further revision, but usually authors revise their papers using the comments and suggestions from reviewers.

After revising the manuscript, the author returns it to the editor, who in turn may read the changes and make a final acceptance decision without another external review. If substantial changes were made in the manuscript or the author was directed to revise and resubmit it, the reviewers critique the revised version and make recommendations to the editor. This revision process continues until the paper is accepted for publication.

EDITORIAL DECISIONS

Not every paper sent to a journal is accepted, nor should it be; this maintains the quality of the journal and meets readers' needs. Rejection rates vary across journals and may be as high as 50% to 90% for prominent journals (Huth, 1999). Some journals receive a large number of manuscripts, significantly more than could be published within a reasonable time frame and, therefore, reject many of these papers. Other journals have fewer submissions and work with authors in revising their papers until acceptable for publication.

Editors monitor the number of papers accepted for publication to avoid a backlog of papers accepted but not published. Journals are allotted a predetermined number of pages for each issue by the publisher. Because of the cost, only these pages are allowed. Therefore, the editor plans which manuscripts to include in each issue, estimating the number to accept so that the time between acceptance and publication is not unreasonable. A delay in publishing accepted papers hinders disseminating new knowledge to readers, and when too much time elapses, papers may need to be updated. Some backlog, though, is needed so that a sufficient number of papers is available for each issue and to allow for fluctuations in submissions without creating a delay in publication.

Criteria for Acceptance of Manuscripts

The criteria used by editors to decide whether to accept a manuscript vary by journal, but Huth (1999, p. 258) identified five general criteria used by most editors in making this decision:

1. Relevance of the paper to the journal's goals and audience
2. Importance of the content for readers
3. Whether the content is new and innovative
4. Extent and validity of evidence to support the conclusions of the paper
5. Usefulness to the journal considering other topics published in it.

The editor also considers the number of papers on the same or similar topics that already have been accepted. It is unlikely that the editor will accept too many articles on similar topics because of the need to publish new content for readers. If the author is notified that the paper is rejected, the backlog of papers may have been an influencing factor, and the rejection may have less to do with the paper's quality and relevance for readers than the backlog of manuscripts.

Types of Editorial Decisions

Three main types of decisions can be made by the editor based on the editor's own review and suggestions from reviewers: (1) accept for publication, (2) revise and resubmit, and (3) reject.

Accept for Publication

Decisions to accept for publication may involve an acceptance with no revisions or limited ones, or a tentative acceptance pending revision. An acceptance without revisions is rare; even if the paper is accepted for publication because of its important and timely content, it is likely that the author will need to make some changes to strengthen it. The author should make these revisions, or provide a rationale for not making them, and return the paper as soon as possible to the editor. The editor may have space to include the paper in an upcoming issue; if not, the paper will have a better chance of being published sooner.

Other acceptances are provisional, with the final decision resting on whether the author revises the manuscript to reflect the changes suggested by the editor and reviewers. Changes might be needed in the content, for example, adding or deleting content, preparing or omitting a table, or including a new section of content; or, the changes might be in the writing style and format. As with acceptance decisions, the author should revise the paper without delay.

Revise and Resubmit

The second type of decision possible is to revise and resubmit for another review. When authors are asked to revise and resubmit the manuscript, it suggests that the paper has merit and would be strengthened by revision. Although revision does not guarantee acceptance, there is interest by the editor and reviewers in the paper and its message. Therefore, the author should take the time to revise the paper as recommended. Again, the author should not delay in resubmitting it.

Reject

The third editorial decision is a rejection. Perhaps the content was not new, and the author missed this in the literature review. The journal might have recently published a series of articles on the same or a similar topic or accepted a paper with the same theme. The content may be too specialized or not specialized enough for readers of the journal or may be of limited interest to readers. The organization of the paper and writing style may be unclear. These are only a few of many reasons for a rejection.

Authors should never regard a rejection as a "personal affront" (McConnell, 1999, p. 83). A manuscript may not be suitable for a publication for many reasons, and the feedback from the editor and reviewers gives the author information about why the paper was rejected. Many well-written papers are rejected because the content and focus do not reflect the needs of the readers, and the paper would be better suited for a different journal and audience. When the reasons for rejection relate to the quality of the writing and development of the content, the author should get editorial assistance in revising the paper and should ask colleagues to critique the content.

The author should evaluate the comments made by the editor and reviewers because these may provide a basis for revising the paper and submitting it to another journal. The second or third journal may be a better fit for the content and writing style, or these journals may have fewer submissions and accept more papers than did the first journal to which the paper was sent. Huth (1999) suggested that another journal of lesser reputation or with more specialized content may readily accept the paper. In revising the paper and submitting it to a different journal, remember to reformat it to fit the journal requirements, including the reference format, writing style, and page limits, so that it appears to be written for that journal.

This revision and resubmission process can be continued until the manuscript is accepted or the author determines that no further revisions are possible. The author might try a nonrefereed journal or newsletter as an option for publication.

MANUSCRIPT REVISION

Authors should understand the review process. Few papers are accepted without some revision. Generally, manuscripts need to be revised whether they are accepted for publication, tentatively accepted pending revision, or need a major revision before resubmission. If the paper is not rejected, the author should revise it using the feedback from the editor and reviewers and resubmit it to the journal within the deadline specified by the editor.

Authors should adhere to this deadline because some editors may accept the manuscript when returned or, if the modifications were substantial, will send it back to the same reviewers (Day, 1998). If the criticisms made by the reviewers were resolved, an acceptance decision is more likely. If the deadline is not met, the revised version of the paper may be treated as a new manuscript and sent to a different set of reviewers (Davidhizar & Bechtel, 1999). The new reviewers may have alternate suggestions for revision and opinions about its acceptance. It is best to avoid this situation by not delaying in resubmitting the paper.

Swartz (1999) suggested that many of the requested revisions occur because authors send manuscripts without giving enough thought to the audience and clarity of expression. Authors may write too quickly, relying on a good review and the editor's comments to revise the paper rather than writing it well for the original submission.

A good review suggests changes that the author should consider. The comments from reviewers are intended as constructive criticism, and usually their questions point out areas where revision is needed. The author can respond by revising the paper as suggested or can provide a rationale as to why those changes are not appropriate.

Purcell, Donovan, and Davidoff (1998) examined changes made in manuscripts during the editorial process. They studied the types of changes that manuscripts undergo as a result of peer review and revisions suggested to authors. Manuscripts were revised because of five types of problems: (1) too much information, (2) too little information, (3) inaccurate information, (4) misplaced information, and (5) structural problems, such as when a table was used instead of text.

Not all suggested revisions have to be made in the paper, but the author should justify why changes were not made rather than sending the paper back without the suggested revisions. The author should indicate which revisions would not strengthen the paper and provide a rationale. Manske (1997) directed authors to provide a "reasonable rebuttal to the criticism" if warranted (p. 771). Sometimes, the proposed revisions would not strengthen the paper, but they also might give the author a clue as to which areas of the paper are not clearly written or have missing information.

Letter to Send With Revision

In revising the paper, the author should prepare a letter to accompany the revised version of the paper that outlines each revision suggested and made in the paper and explains why certain changes were not made. The letter should indicate the following:

- Each change proposed by the editor and reviewers
- Specific revisions made in response to each of these proposed changes
- Location of the revisions, for example, the exact page number, paragraph, and sentence (or line) where the revision is located
- Changes proposed and not made in the manuscript, accompanied by a rationale.

Display 13.1 provides examples of letters to submit with a revised manuscript that summarize the changes suggested and subsequently made in the paper. The letters also give examples of how to respond to suggestions that were not made in the revised version of the paper. The changes suggested by reviewers can be labeled by the reviewer's number, for instance, reviewer #1, so that it is clear to the editor who had suggested the revision.

Conflicting Reviewer Comments

Reviewers sometimes might give conflicting advice to authors. One reviewer may suggest expanding a content area, whereas another recommends eliminating it. As a result, the author is unsure how to revise the paper to improve it. The first step is to reread the comments to confirm that they are conflicting. It may be that both reviewers identified a problem in the text or figures even though their suggestions for revision are different. If the author is asked to expand a content area by one reviewer and to delete it by the other, it may be that the paper is not clearly written in that section; the conflicting comments suggest some problem with that area of content.

The author should avoid the tendency to leave the writing in its original form (Johnson, 1996). If neither of the reviewers suggests a change to improve the manuscript, the author should decide how best to revise it.

Decision Not to Revise

There are times, however, when authors cannot modify the paper sufficiently to reflect the concerns of the editor and reviewers. In these situations, the author might send it to another journal or rewrite the paper for a different type of publication, for example, modifying a research report for submission to a clinical journal that emphasizes patient care rather than the research itself, describing how the instrument was developed and validated, and preparing an integrated literature review for a publication. At some point, the author may need to abandon the attempt to publish work.

In other situations, the author may decide not to take the time to substantially revise the manuscript to address the editor's and reviewers' concerns. This decision should be made carefully by weighing the alternatives of revis-

DISPLAY 13.1	Sample Letters With Revised Manuscript

EXAMPLE 1

Manuscript: #01-74 Experiences of Students in Pediatric Nursing Clinical Courses

Revisions Proposed (page numbers refer to original manuscript)	Revisions Made (page numbers refer to revised manuscript)
Editor:	
Change first heading of abstract to Issues and Purpose and include statement of issue that prompted research.	Heading revised and statement added (p. 2, paragraph 1)
Discuss rationale for factor analysis considering sample size of 75.	Factor analysis was done in the original study with 416 students. Paragraph on factor analysis revised to clarify this (p. 10, paragraph 2, sentence 1).
Reviewer 1:	
Add ``qualitative portion" to description of Pagana questionnaire in abstract (p. 2).	Sentence was revised (p. 2): "Students (n = 75) completed a modified Pagana Clinical Stress Questionnaire (CSQ), *which collected both quantitative and qualitative data,* at the end of their pediatric nursing clinical course."
On pp. 3–4, include edits on text.	Included as suggested.
On p. 5, include statement as to why pediatric nursing was more stressful to students (in prior studies).	Sentence included on p. 5, paragraph 1, sentence 2.
On p. 7, line 4, add "compared with students in other clinical courses."	Added (see p. 7, line 11)
On p. 8 (and on p. 9, paragraph 3, line 1; p. 11, paragraph 1, line 1), were stress and challenge measured as separate variables? How did instrument collect qualitative data (also questioned on p. 10, paragraph 3, line 1, and on p. 15, line 3)?	Stress and challenge measured by individual Likert scales; six open-ended questions collected qualitative data. Description of instrument revised (p. 8, paragraph 2)
P. 8, Procedure: Were instruments anonymous?	Instruments were anonymous; no identifying information was collected. Added on p. 8, paragraph 1, line 3. Also added to text as recommended (p. 9, paragraph 2, line 3)
Add table with data.	Table 1 added (p. 19)
P. 10, paragraph 2, last sentence: How did these findings compare with other group?	Consistent with nonpediatric courses; added (p. 10, last sentence)
On p. 11, were there any relationships between challenge and emotions?	No (added on p. 11, paragraph 3, last sentence)
P. 12, paragraph 2, line 2: Move M and SD to follow "curriculum."	Moved (p. 12, paragraph 2, line 4)
P. 12, last paragraph: How were the data obtained on factors that facilitate and inhibit learning?	These data were collected with the other qualitative data. Revision of the description of instrument clarifies the different types of information collected (see p. 8, paragraph 2). Sentence on qualitative data now reads: "In Part 2 of the CSQ, qualitative data were

(continued)

Sample Letters With Revised Manuscript *(Continued)*

Revisions Proposed (page numbers refer to original manuscript)	Revisions Made (page numbers refer to revised manuscript)
	collected through six open-ended questions, which enabled the participant to describe the types of stresses and challenges they experienced in clinical practice and factors that facilitated and inhibited their learning."
Reviewer 2: In abstract and on p. 11, only report *P* (not *r*).	Prefer to include the actual correlations with the *P* values. Rationale from *AMA Manual of Style* (9th ed.): Correlations should be reported with coefficient followed by significance (eg, *r* = 0.61, *P* < .001; p. 541)
P. 3, paragraph 2, line 7: Change patient to patients.	Done
On p. 4, line 5, add n.	n = 416; added (p. 4, paragraph 1, line 3)
P. 4, paragraph 1: Delete last sentence.	Deleted
On pp. 4–5, move paragraph 2 to p. 5 and sentences on Kleehammer et al. study (p. 5, lines 4–6) to p. 4.	Revisions made as suggested, with minor editing
P. 5, paragraph 2, lines 4 and 5: Were the goals the patterns found in ethnographic data analysis?	Author of article uses "goals"
On p. 6, paragraph 1, change "area" to "theme."	"Area" of stress changed to "theme"
P. 6, paragraphs 2 and 3: Consider moving these two paragraphs to earlier section of literature with other quantitative studies.	The first set of studies reported in literature review (pp. 4–5) relate to pediatric experiences of *students* (including both quantitative and qualitative studies). Research on p. 6 is on pediatric *nurses* (including both types of studies). Therefore, literature review was not reorganized.
P. 7, line 1: Change "Several studies" to "The studies noted here."	Done
P. 8, last paragraph: Why were deans contacted?	To gain access to institution and identify contact person for distribution of instruments
Results: Add table.	Table 1 added (p. 19)
On p. 13, delete last 2 sentences.	Sentences deleted
P. 15: Add sentence written on text.	Sentence added and all other editing done as recommended (p. 15, last paragraph)

(continued)

| DISPLAY 13.1 | **Sample Letters With Revised Manuscript** *(Continued)* |

EXAMPLE 2

Manuscript #2001-06038 Parents' Views of Quality Health Care
Revisions Suggested and Made in Manuscript:

Editor

1. Add a table on demographic data, comparing the two groups: Table added (see p. 16, Table 1).
2. Include a list of pertinent web sites: Added (see pp. 18–19).

Reviewer 1

1. Weakness of study is lack of information about consumers: Findings added in text (see pp. 6–7, lines 12–16). Table added that presents demographic data (see p. 16, Table 1).
2. Add information on consumers such as age, educational level, marital status, views of nursing care of children: Ages of consumers (see p. 7, lines 2–7); educational level (see pp. 6–7, lines 12–13 and p. 16, Table 1); marital status (see p. 7, lines 8–10 and p. 16, Table 1). Other demographic data presented on p. 7, lines 10–12. Views of nursing care of children are part of the Results.
3. Indicators not specific to care of children but, nevertheless, are general enough to provide information on perception of quality; investigator should have completed a pilot study: Paragraph on this limitation was rewritten (see p. 11, lines 3–4). Pilot study was completed but did not reveal this limitation (see p. 6, paragraph 1).

Reviewer 2

1. How were subjects identified and accessed?: Sentence added on p. 5, paragraph 2, sentence 3.
2. Did the study go through IRB?: Yes, sentence added on p. 5 (line 8).
3. In terms of the Quality Health Care Questionnaire (QHCQ), is most of the literature used to identify indicators (for instrument) included in reference list of manuscript? Is so, add statement to this effect: No, the literature used to identify indicators for the QHCQ is much more extensive than that reported in manuscript. Therefore, statement was not added.
4. Indicators and factors used interchangeably in this section: Differences between the indicators and factors are explained on pp. 5–6 (lines 9–11). No revisions were made in this section.

ing the paper for a journal showing some interest versus sending it to another journal where there may be minimal interest in its content. If the author decides not to revise and return the manuscript, the editor should be notified so that records can be kept current.

TIME FRAME FOR DECISION

If the editor decides not to review the manuscript, the author will be notified of this decision within a few weeks. The length of time varies widely for peer reviewers to critique a manuscript, for the editor to compile and summarize the reviews, and for an editorial decision to be made. Many journals ask peer reviewers to complete their critiques within 3 weeks, but not everyone is able to meet this deadline. Reviewers have competing demands, and it sometimes takes longer than anticipated.

The earliest that the author would be notified about the decision on whether to publish the manuscript is approximately 8 weeks after it is submitted to the journal. Some editors make their editorial decisions more quickly than others, but generally it takes at least 8 weeks to complete the review process and notify the author of the publication decision. If the author has not heard by 12 weeks, the author should contact to editor to inquire about the status of the review.

 ## LENGTH OF TIME TO PUBLICATION

Journals vary in their backlogs of accepted manuscripts waiting to be published. Some journals have a backlog of 1 or 2 years, whereas others may publish the manuscript 6 months after the final version is accepted.

 ## HONORARIUM

Most scientific journals do not reimburse the author when a manuscript is accepted for publication. Unlike magazines for consumers, who generally pay authors for an accepted paper, most nursing and health care journals do not give an honorarium. When they do, though, this often is specified in the author guidelines. For example, *AORN Journal* indicates that an honorarium will be sent to the author after publication, as well as a copy of the issue and reprints of it (AORN, 2001). *Nursing 2001* pays authors approximately $50 per printed page. When the article is published, the editor sends an honorarium to the primary author plus complimentary copies of the issue in which the article appears (Nursing 2001, 2001).

Most journals provide complimentary copies of the issue in which the article appears and reprints of it. Reprints also can be purchased if the author needs more; usually, these must be ordered at the page proof stage, not when the article is published.

SUMMARY

The primary responsibilities of the editor are to solicit manuscripts, work with authors to develop their ideas into manuscripts that are suitable for publication, assess the quality of manuscripts submitted to the journal, decide on manuscripts to publish based on recommendations from the reviewers, and edit manuscripts. Editors work with authors, editorial board members, manuscript reviewers, and the production editor. In addition to the editor, some journals also have a managing editor, who is a paid professional responsible for the administrative details associated with processing the manuscripts from submission through publication.

Journals rely on external or peer reviewers, sometimes called referees, to read and critically judge the manuscripts submitted to the journal. Peer reviewers are experts in the topic of the manuscript; they are considered "peers" of the author because they have similar expertise allowing them to critique the paper. Peer reviewers give expert opinions about the manuscript and make recommendations to the editor concerning its acceptance.

Many peer reviewed journals use a process of blind review in which submitted manuscripts are sent to reviewers with the identity of the author and institution concealed. The editor removes the title page and conceals other identifying information. The principle behind sending a "blinded" copy, free of identifying information, is that there is less chance of bias.

Reviewers also are unknown to the author. When reviews are returned to the author, the identities of the reviewers are masked so that the author does not know who read the paper. With this anonymity, reviewers are free to evaluate a paper honestly and without fear of repercussions from the author if they give a negative review. It is believed that these reviews are fairer.

When the manuscript arrives in the editorial office of the journal, it is given a number, which is used throughout the review process to track the manuscript. Not all manuscripts are sent out for review. If the manuscript is not relevant for the journal, the editor is likely to return the manuscript to the author without its being reviewed. The manuscript also may be returned to the author if it is incomplete or does not conform to the journal requirements.

After the editor determines the suitability of the manuscript for the journal, the review process begins. The editor decides who should review the manuscript based on who has the expertise to evaluate it. At least two reviews usually are completed for each paper. The results of the peer review then are sent to the author with the editorial decision on whether the paper is accepted, should be revised and resubmitted, or is rejected. The reviews provide data for the editor to use in making an acceptance decision and feedback for authors in revising the paper to strengthen it.

The criteria used by editors to decide whether to accept a manuscript vary by journal, but most editors use the following general criteria to make this decision: (1) relevance of the paper for the journal, (2) importance of the content, (3) whether the content is new and innovative, (4) validity of evidence to support the conclusions of the paper, (5) usefulness to the journal considering other topics published in it, and (6) the number of papers on the same or similar topics that already have been accepted.

Three main types of decisions can be made by the editor based on the editor's own review and suggestions from reviewers: (1) accept for publication, (2) revise and resubmit, and (3) reject. Decisions to accept for publication may involve an acceptance with no revisions or limited ones, or a tentative acceptance pending revision. An acceptance without revisions is rare; even if the paper is accepted for publication because of its important and timely content, the author usually needs to make some changes to strengthen it. Other acceptances are provisional, with the final decision resting on whether the author revises the manuscript to reflect the changes suggested by the editor and reviewers.

The second type of decision possible is revise and resubmit for another review. When authors are asked to revise and resubmit the manuscript, it suggests that the paper has merit and would be strengthened by a revision. The third editorial decision is a rejection.

A good review suggests changes that the author should consider. The author can respond by revising the paper as suggested or can provide a rationale as to why those changes are not appropriate. Not all suggested changes have to be made in the paper, but the author should justify why changes were not made rather than sending back the paper without the suggested revisions. The author should prepare a letter to accompany the revised version of the paper that explains each revision suggested and made in the paper, as well as changes not made and why.

When the manuscript is accepted for publication, the paper moves into the next phase. The author has some responsibilities here, such as answering queries and correcting page proofs, but most of the work is done by the publisher.

REFERENCES

AORN. (1999). AORN Journal: Author guidelines. [On-line]. Available: *http://www.aorn.org/journal/guidelines.htm*. Accessed June 17, 2001.

Baggs, J.G. (1999). The value of the blind review process: Is blindness best? *Research in Nursing & Health, 22*, 93–94.

Barnum, B.S. (1995). *Writing and getting published: A primer for nurses.* New York: Springer.

Blackwell, A.H. (2000, June 2). Reviews of journal manuscripts: Nasty, petty, arrogant. *The Chronicle of Higher Education, 46*(39), B10.

Blancett, S.S. (1997). Nursing journal leadership. *Nursing Administration Quarterly, 22*(1), 16–22.

Davidhizar, R., & Bechtel, G.A. (1999). Avoiding publication delays: Author and editor responsibilities. *Nurse Author & Editor, 9*(4), 1–4, 7.

Day, R.A. (1998). *How to write and publish a scientific paper* (5th ed.). Phoenix, AZ: Oryx Press.

Earnshaw, J.J., Farndon, J.R., Guillou, P.J., Johnson, C.D., Murie, J.A., & Murray, G.D. (2000). A comparison of reports from referees chosen by authors or journal editors in the peer review process. *Annals of the Royal College of Surgeons of England, 82*(Suppl. 4), 133–135.

Fondiller, S.H. (1999). *The writer's workbook* (2nd ed.). Sudbury, MA: Jones & Bartlett.

Huth, E.J. (1999). *Writing and publishing in medicine* (3rd ed.). Baltimore: Lippincott Williams & Wilkins.

International Committee of Medical Journal Editors. (1997). Uniform requirements for manuscripts submitted to biomedical journals. *Annals of Internal Medicine, 126*, 36–47. Available at: http://www.icmj.org/.

Johnson, S. H. (1996). Dealing with conflicting reviewers' comments. *Nurse Author & Editor, 6*(4), 1–3.

Justice, A.C., Cho, M.K., Winker, M.A., Berlin, J.A., Rennie, D., & PEER Investigators. (1998). Does masking author identity improve peer review quality? *Journal of the American Medical Association, 280*, 240–242.

Kronick, D.A. (1990). Peer review in the 18th-century scientific journalism. *Journal of the American Medical Association, 263*, 1321–1322.

Manske, P. R. (1997). A review of peer review. *Journal of Hand Surgery, 22A*, 767–771.

McConnell, C.R. (1999). From idea to print: Writing for a professional journal. *Health Care Supervisor, 17*(3), 72–85.

Nursing 2001. (2001). Author guidelines. [On-line]. Available: *http://www.springnet.com/jrdescr/jrn-d41.htm#10*. Accessed June 17, 2001.

Purcell, G.P., Donovan, S.L., & Davidoff, F. (1998). Changes to manuscripts during the editorial process. *Journal of the American Medical Association, 280*, 227–228.

Rothwell, P.M., & Martyn, C.N. (2000). Reproducibility of peer review in clinical neuroscience: Is agreement between reviewers any greater than would be expected by chance alone? *Brain*, 123 (Pt. 9), 1964–1969.

Swartz, K. (1999). Peer-reviewed journals and quality. *Inquiry, 36*, 119–121.

Thomas, S.P. (1998). The long journey to publication: Some thoughts on the journal review process. *Issues in Mental Health Nursing, 19*, 415–418.

van Rooyen, S., Godlee, F., Evans, S., Smith, R., & Black, N. (1998). Effect of blinding and unmasking on the quality of peer review. *Journal of the American Medical Association, 280*, 234–237.

Yankauer, A. (1991). How blind is blind review? *American Journal of Public Health, 81*, 843–845.

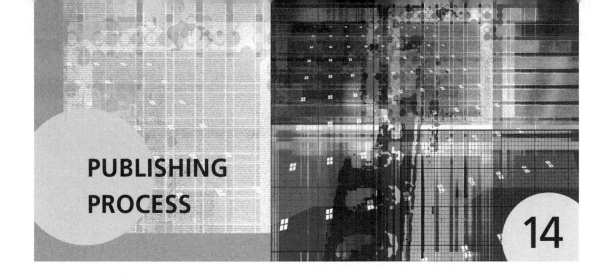

PUBLISHING PROCESS

14

When the manuscript is accepted for publication, the paper moves into the publishing phase. The author has some responsibilities here, such as answering queries and correcting page proofs, but most of the work is done by the journal's publisher or by the group or individual responsible for the publication. The manuscript is edited for clarity and consistency with the journal style and format; the copy editor usually has questions for the author about the manuscript. These questions, or queries, must be answered and the proofs must be reviewed to confirm the accuracy of the content after editing and to check other details.

This chapter describes the publishing process, which begins with the acceptance of the paper and moves through its publication. Publishers have different ways of handling the editing phase of the manuscript and the forms of the manuscript used for author proofing. Although the publishing process is described here, the author should recognize that this differs across journals. When the paper is published by an organization or individual, the process may vary from what is described in this chapter.

WHAT HAPPENS NEXT?

The time from acceptance of the paper to its publication varies with the journal, depending on its backlog and other factors, such as the relationship of the topic to that of other papers waiting to be published or the focus of a particular issue. It could take from a minimum of 3 or 4 months to 1 year or longer before the paper is published (McConnell, 1999). When the editor decides on the issue in which the paper will appear, the author is notified of this and when to expect the edited manuscript or page proofs to review.

In this stage of publication, the author reviews the edited manuscript or page proofs, answers questions raised by the copy editor, corrects any errors in the paper as a result of the editing or formatting, and checks other details such as word divisions, accuracy of tables, and accuracy of author information. Even though the author reviewed the manuscript thoroughly before sending the final version, the paper has since been edited, and the author needs to verify that the changes made during editing did not alter the intended meaning. This is the last chance for the author to find errors in the paper before its publication.

The author used to receive a version of the paper that was set in type and then printed on paper. Often, these were in the form of galley proofs—printouts of the document with large margins, allowing the author to read what was printed and record comments or indicate errors. This system was important when journals were printed with lead type (Huth, 1999).

The purpose of the author's review of the typeset pages, similar to current publishing, was to identify errors and correct them. After the corrections were made in the galley proofs, they were assembled into pages. Authors often were not asked to review the page proofs; this was done by the publisher.

Most of these steps now are computerized. Authors generally submit the final version as an electronic file, which is used to develop the proofs of the article. Authors still need to review the edited manuscript or page proofs carefully, though, because the edited version may have altered the intended meaning, and other errors may be present.

Generally, there is a limited period of time—for some journals, only 48 hours—for the author to read and correct the proofs of the manuscript. The author should adhere to this time frame. Otherwise, the article may be printed as is with any errors present. Authors should notify the editor if there is a change in address or if an alternate address should be used for sending the page proofs, such as in the case of faculty who may not be at the school of nursing during a particular semester.

FORMATS FOR AUTHOR REVIEW

Before publication, a copy editor revises the paper for clarity and for format so that it conforms to the style of the journal. This may include rewriting some of the text to make it clearer, correcting grammatical problems, reformatting tables, or modifying references. The editing, though, may have inadvertently changed some of the meaning. The author is responsible for identifying this when reviewing the edited manuscript. There also may be questions or queries for the author about the content, references, tables, and illustrations.

Edited Manuscript

Some journals send an edited version of the manuscript to the author that shows the original text with the corrections. The author should read the edited version carefully, noting any errors or changes that are needed, because this may be the only chance to correct the paper before publication. Some journals send only this copy to proofread and indicate approval.

Page Proofs

With other journals, the author receives the edited paper in the form of page proofs, which are similar to the pages of the journal and incorporate the copy editor's revisions. Some journals send both the edited copy and the page proofs.

 ## PROOFING THE MANUSCRIPT

Authors are sent an edited version of their manuscript or page proofs for two purposes: to check for errors and answer queries about it. Errors may result from the changes made by the copy editor or from reformatting the manuscript to conform to the journal's style.

In correcting these errors, the author can insert text by printing it above the line where it belongs or in the margin next to it and then placing a caret (∧) under the line of text to indicate where it should be inserted. If the text to be inserted does not fit in the margin, it can be typed on a separate piece of paper and attached to the edited pages with a caret indicating where to insert it. To delete text, the author can cross it out with a horizontal line.

Other marks used to indicate corrections on the edited version or page proofs are called proofreaders' marks. A list of these is found in Appendix 2. These marks are universal.

Day (1998) recommended that authors note errors twice: once at the point where it occurs, and once in the margin next to it. This double-marking system assures the author that the corrections will be noticed.

At this point in publication, the author cannot rewrite the text except for what is necessary to correct the errors. The paper was accepted as submitted in the final version, after peer review, so rewriting is not appropriate at this stage. If the content has changed since the paper was accepted, this should be discussed with the editor rather than modifying the page proofs. Changes at this point in the publishing process are expensive and, therefore, should focus only on the accuracy of the content.

Answering Queries

The author must answer each query raised by the copy editor. Often, this is easily done by checking a revision, inserting text, modifying a reference, or revising the table or text so that they are consistent. Some queries require an explanation, which the author can write in the margin or provide as an attachment. The author should make it clear what revisions were made in the manuscript in response to the editor's queries. If unable to answer a question, this also should be noted.

Areas to Proof

What should the author check when proofing the edited version or page proofs? First, the main goal is to ensure that there are no errors in the content. Sometimes, a minor editorial revision changes the meaning of the sentence, and this is the author's only chance to correct the paper before publication. The author should confirm that the content is accurate, the changes made by the editor did not alter the meaning, nothing essential was omitted from the paper, and the tables and illustrations are numbered correctly, with the corresponding numbers in the text.

In proofreading the paper, the author should compare the original copy sent to the editor with the page proofs. A colleague can read the original copy while the author checks the proofs.

Second, the author should check for spelling and grammatical errors. Even though this was a done in preparing the final version, a misspelled word might not have been noticed, and words correctly spelled might have been used incorrectly, such as rational for rationale. The author should not rely on the copy editor for identifying these errors. The spelling of authors' names, their credentials, their positions, and the contact information of the corresponding author should be verified. The author should check that the title of the article is correct, including the spelling.

The author also should pay attention to how words are divided. To align the right margin of the text, some words may need to be divided. The author should check that these divisions of words are correct and make sense. Generally, a break in the word can be checked in the dictionary if the author is unsure.

Third, the author should review the abbreviations, numerical values in the text and tables, statistical results, references, tables, and illustrations. Errors may have occurred when these were formatted for the style of the journal. For research articles, the author should verify that the numbers used to report the findings are the same in the abstract, text, tables, and figures, and that no data are missing. The author should check carefully numbers with decimals, P values, and statistics. The copy editor may have made changes in how the statistics are presented to conform to the journal's style, so the author needs to review these for any errors.

The names of authors cited in the text should be compared with the reference list. If numbers are used for the citations, these should match the correct reference.

For some journals, tables require substantial reformatting, so tables in the proofs should be checked against the original (Byrne, 1998). Each column and row should be examined, paying attention to whether the numbers are accurate and are lined up properly. Footnotes from the original copy may be changed to use the journal's symbols, so the author should verify that footnotes are included and are correct.

The proofs of illustrations should be examined carefully to ensure that they will be clear when published. The author provides the quality control in the reproduction of illustrations, and it is best to discuss concerns with the editor before publication rather than after (Day, 1998). Titles of the tables and illustrations also should be reviewed.

Display 14.1 is a checklist for authors to use when reading page proofs. Authors should not take this step lightly because the author is responsible for identifying and correcting errors before the paper is printed (Huth, 1999). Johnson (1998) suggested that checking the page proofs is the most important step in the publishing process because errors here "end up in print" (p. 1).

 ## CITING PAPERS "IN PRESS"

Manuscripts accepted for publication by the journal can be cited as "in press" (American Medical Association, 1997; Huth, 1999). Once authors have reviewed page proofs and have been notified of the publication date, volume, and issue, they can add this information to the reference if it is cited in another paper they are writing.

 ## REPRINTS

After reviewing and correcting the page proofs, the author has some assurance that the manuscript will be printed without errors and in the issue indicated by the editor. Generally, the page proofs are reviewed a few months before publication. Many journals send forms for ordering reprints with the page proofs. If the author is interested in having reprints to distribute to colleagues or students, they should be ordered when the page proofs are reviewed or when the author receives the information about reprints. After the journal is published, reprints may be more expensive or may not be available. Thus, authors should decide early if they want reprints.

Proofing Checklist

Pay attention to all details when proofing. If necessary, read through the pages several times until all of these aspects have been checked. Use this checklist to proof your manuscript before submitting it for publication and again to check page proofs.

✔ All content is double-checked and is accurate and correct, including any number, physiologic concept, drugs, drug dosage, medical treatments, nursing interventions, nursing theories, references, tables, and figures.

✔ All proper names in the article either have a reference to the source or the author has obtained written permission to use the name in the article. (Proper names include the name of the person, hospital, company, product, or other proper or proprietary name.)

✔ All company or product names have the appropriate trademark or registered mark attached to that name as required by federal trademark law.

✔ Grammar is correct, including sentence structure, punctuation, spelling, and subject–verb agreement.

✔ Drug names are listed by generic name, and all generic names are in lowercase letters.

✔ All drug dosages, actions, and side effects are correct and have references to the source.

✔ All written permissions for using or adapting copyrighted material have been received, and the credit line on the material agrees with the credit line specified by the copyright holder in the permit.

✔ All abbreviations are spelled out the first time used.

✔ All specific statements, including numbers, percents, dosages, quotes, side effects, product or company names, and orders, have reference numbers at the end of that sentence to reference the original source of the information.

✔ All references are complete.

✔ Typing, grammar, and headings have been proofed and are correct.

✔ Hyphens placed at the end of lines in which split words appear are in correct locations.

✔ Page flow is correct, where text reads correctly from one page to the next.

✔ Text has no typographical, accuracy, or grammatical problems.

✔ Large-font words are correct, including titles and headings.

✔ Art, figures, tables, and illustrations are correct, including titles, headings, text, captions, and footnotes.

✔ Items in a bulleted list are consistent within the list.

✔ Use of initial capital letters is consistent in lists, tables, and headings (eg, no initial capital in one item and lowercase in another).

✔ If a case study is included, the name and all identifying characteristics have been changed for confidentiality, and a case disclaimer is included.

✔ The author's background is accurate and includes the information used by the target publication.

✔ Once you are finished, set it aside for 1 hour, then glance at the overall major components again, such as titles, captions, and tables.

From Johnson, S.H. (1998). The proofing challenge: Finding hidden errors. *Nurse Author & Editor, 8*(3), 3. Copyright 1998 Hall Johnson Consulting. Reproduced with permission. For further use contact the publisher at 9737 West Ohio Avenue, Lakewood, CO 80226; NurseAuthorMail@aol.com.

The number of reprints to order is up to the author, but it is best to over-order. Generally, the more reprints ordered, the less expensive they are for the author.

Some authors may want to distribute copies of their paper before it is published or post it on the Web. However, remember that the copyright was transferred to the publisher, and any earlier publication of the paper would need to be consistent with the conditions in the copyright transfer. The author should discuss this with the editor.

After the article is published, the author will receive a limited number of complimentary copies of the journal. Complimentary copies are not sent to co-authors, so the first or corresponding author is responsible for distributing copies to them.

CORRECTIONS AND RETRACTIONS

If the author discovers after an article is published that there were errors in the data reported or the conclusions reached, the author should contact the editor and submit a letter correcting the information. A correction, or erratum, of part of the work will be published in a later issue of the journal (International Committee of Medical Journal Editors [ICMJE], 1997).

If there is scientific fraud, however, the paper should be retracted (ICMJE, 1997). The author should send a letter, signed by co-authors, to the editor requesting a retraction and indicating the reasons. The retraction will be published in a subsequent issue of the journal. If the paper is not yet published, the editor usually allows the author to withdraw it. Along the same line, if the author determines later that a co-author published the same data in another paper without indicating this in the current article, a letter should be sent to the editor, who will note this as a repetitive publication.

SUMMARY

The publication stage provides an opportunity for the author to review the edited manuscript or page proofs, answer questions raised by the copy editor, correct any errors in the paper as a result of the editing or formatting, and check other details such as word divisions, accuracy of tables, and accuracy of author information. Although the author reviewed the manuscript thoroughly before sending the final copy, the paper has since been edited, and the author needs to verify that the changes made during editing did not alter the intended meaning. This is the last chance for the author to find errors in the paper before its publication. There also may be questions or queries for the author about the text, references, or tables and illustrations.

There is generally a limited period of time for the author to read and correct the proofs of the manuscript, and the author should adhere to this time frame. Otherwise, the article may be printed as is, with any errors present.

Authors should notify the editor if there is any change in address and if an alternate address should be used for sending the page proofs.

In some instances, the author is sent an edited version of the manuscript showing the corrections made in the paper. The edited manuscript displays the original text and each change. With other journals, the author receives the paper in the form of page proofs, which are similar to the pages of the journal and incorporate the copy editor's revisions. Some journals send both the edited copy and the page proofs.

The edited manuscript or page proofs are sent to the author to identify errors, not for rewriting. After correcting the page proofs, the author has some assurance that the manuscript will be printed without errors and in the issue indicated by the editor. Generally, the page proofs are reviewed a few months before publication. Most journals send forms for ordering reprints with the page proofs. When the article is published, the author receives complimentary copies of the journal.

REFERENCES

American Medical Association. (1998). *Manual of style: A guide for authors and editors* (9th ed.). Baltimore: Lippincott Williams & Wilkins.

Byrne, D.W. (1998). *Publishing your medical research paper*. Baltimore: Lippincott Williams & Wilkins.

Day, R.A. (1998). *How to write and publish a scientific paper* (5th ed.). Phoenix, AZ: Oryx Press.

Huth, E.J. (1999). *Writing and publishing in medicine* (3rd ed.). Baltimore: Lippincott Williams & Wilkins.

International Committee of Medical Journal Editors. (1997). Uniform requirements for manuscripts submitted to biomedical journals. *Annals of Internal Medicine, 126*(1), 36–47. Available at: http://www.icmje.org/.

Johnson, S.H. (1998). The proofing challenge: Finding hidden errors. *Nurse Author & Editor, 8*(3), 1–4, 7.

McConnell, C.R. (1999). From idea to print: Writing for a professional journal. *Health Care Supervisor, 17*(3), 72–85.

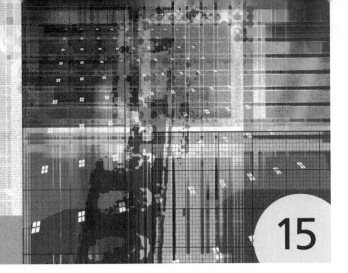

WORLD WIDE WEB AND ELECTRONIC PUBLISHING EARLY EXPERIENCES AND FUTURE TRENDS

15

The Internet and the World Wide Web mark the beginning of an era that will change the world and individuals in ways we cannot conceive of today. We already are experiencing phenomenal change in communication, and windows are opening into worlds unseen by many of us before: other countries, out in space, and beneath the sea. In the arena of electronic publication, the Web opens up possibilities for greater exposure and dissemination of articles and information. It allows for collaborative workspace. It also accommodates different formats for delivering content.

When an article is accepted for publication, the author may find it published on the Web before or after it appears in the printed journal. Some authors may decide to submit an article to a journal published only on-line. This chapter examines current variations in electronic publishing and speculates about what the future may hold for authors in nursing and other health fields.

STAGES OF NEW TECHNOLOGY

This chapter is organized around a framework developed by John Naisbitt (1991) in his book *Megatrends*, originally published in 1984. According to Naisbitt, new technologies progress through three stages:

- Stage 1: Content is moved from an old medium to the new technology and resembles the media that it is replacing.
- Stage 2: People start to exploit the unique features of the new technology, and it moves into a stage where marked improvement and innovation occur.

- Stage 3: New directions and uses are discovered that grow out of the technology itself.

Stage 1: Early Learning Experiences

Most on-line journals began by posting articles on a Web site that had already existed in print. This is how the American Journal of Nursing (AJN) Company began its on-line publishing. AJN Online was funded by a grant from the Division of Nursing (Department of Health and Human Services, Public Health Service) to the AJN Company in 1993. It started as an 800-number dial-up bulletin board service (BBS) and then became available over the Internet in 1994. Suddenly, the Web was there, so in January 1995, AJN moved the content from the BBS and added an entire issue of the journal to the new Web site.

It was not a creative approach but a necessary first step to learn the capabilities of the technology. There were many new discoveries in the process of learning how to use this new technology. An early learning experience involved the insistence of one editor to put the AJN articles on the Web in three columns, just as they appear in print, citing several readability studies supporting this layout. Developers had to create a page in three columns to convince the editor that this approach would not work on a Web page.

The process of getting an article on the Web took longer than expected. Developers could not use the original text files because significant changes had occurred in articles by the time they emerged from the editor's word processor, passed through desk-top publishing, and finally appeared in print. Converting an article back into a format for use on the Web was far from automatic, even with software designed for that purpose. It can take more than 3 hours to get an article of average length ready for display on a Web page.

Another major step was learning to create pages dynamically. This involves storing elements of an article (eg, title, author, abstract, images) in separate database fields instead of using a single, flat file for all the elements of an article.

Most nursing journals began electronic publishing by posting tables of contents, some with abstracts, on the Web, hoping that they would attract new subscribers for the printed journal. Murray and Anthony (1999) referred to these as "webverts" in their discussion of the continuum of electronic publishing. Many journal editors quickly recognized the Web's potential and added interactive features to catch the interest to their readership; for example, they created Web sites of interest to readers of the particular journal and interactive sites with opportunities to pose questions to the authors.

One innovative author, Sparks (1999) of the National Library of Medicine, developed an article on electronic publishing and nursing research for the journal *Nursing Research*. The article was put on-line before it was published in print. In the article, Sparks embedded Uniform Resource Locators with links in her on-line version and conducted an on-line poll, soliciting readers for their opinions on issues related to electronic publishing.

Some of these efforts to use the interactivity of the Web were quickly embraced by readers, and others were largely ignored. For example, AJN tried to stimulate interest in a journal club where readers could discuss each specific article. Authors also were invited to join, but this feature met with limited success and was discontinued.

Continuing Education Offerings

Journals also began offering continuing education (CE) on-line. After reading an article, readers take the CE test electronically, use cybercash to pay for CE processing, and receive instant grading of the CE test, complete with a certificate that can be printed immediately.

A Different Approach: On-Line Journals and 'Zines

Early in Web history, journals began to appear on the Web that never existed in print format. There are several advantages to publishing directly on the Web. Articles can be published quickly. There is no need to wait, and there are no page or space restrictions. Sparks (1999) cited several other advantages. She observed that publication on the Web makes articles accessible worldwide. Search engines automatically add the publication to their databases, and translation software can make the information available in other languages. In addition, Sparks noted that software on web servers can track the use of materials.

The following nursing journals are on-line only. These also are called e-journals, and all are peer reviewed:

- Sigma Theta Tau's *Online Journal of Knowledge Synthesis in Nursing* (OJKSN), at *http://www.stti.iupui.edu/library/ojksn*, first published in December 1993.
- *Australian Electronic Journal of Nursing Education,* at *http://www.csu. edu.au/faculty/health/nurshealth/aejne/index.html*, first published in December 1995.
- *Online Journal of Issues in Nursing* (OJIN) at *http://www.ana.org/ojin/ index.htm*, first published in June 1996.
- *Online Journal of Nursing Informatics* (OJNI), at *http://milkman.cac. psu.edu/dxm12/OJNI.html*, first published in the winter of 1997.

Some articles in on-line journals are in a portable document file (PDF). A PDF file allows the reader to print the file in a format that replicates the print version almost exactly, with columns and embedded tables. Printing a PDF file requires a software package called Acrobat Reader, which may be downloaded at no cost. Journals make large bodies of text available in PDF format to allow readers to print it and read off-line. Early studies document that it takes 25% to 30% longer to read text from a computer screen.

In the United Kingdom, *Nursing Standard* (*http://www.nursing-standard. co.uk*) pioneered a hybrid approach. They became the first weekly nursing e-journal and combined a selection of items from the printed journal with a unique on-line section (Murray & Anthony, 1999).

'Zines are different from on-line journals. Some are delivered by electronic mail (email), some are posted on the Web, and some appear in both forms. They generally are not peer reviewed as are on-line journals. Most 'zines contain "what's new" features rather than scholarly information, with much of the content focusing on new information on the Web. Some 'zines are little more than email alerts that hype what's new on their own Web site.

Distinguishing Between Portals and Electronic Journals

The term "portal" refers to a Web site that offers a broad array of resources and services. Generally, a portal has a significant amount of content and also is a point of access to other Web sites with content that is likely to be of interest to their users. Portals contain community-building areas, such as forums and chat discussions. Most provide email, personalization features, and e-commerce opportunities.

The first portals on the Web were America Online and the major search engines. NursingCenter.com is a vertical portal for nurses with a goal of providing a wide variety of information to nurses in all areas of practice, education, and research. It was never intended to be an electronic publishing site. From the first glimmer of an idea, the site was conceived as an information resource. The first content that appeared on the BBS site was forums, followed by databases. Currently, most of the information on the Web site comes from journal content, but each journal that resides on NursingCenter.com defines and shapes its own on-line presence and identity. NursingCenter.com is a vehicle for access to many sources of information.

Other professional portals of interest to nurses include the American Nurses Association Web site (*http://www.nursingworld.org*) and Medscape (*http://www.medscape.com*). More are appearing daily. Many license content from printed journals for some articles and also use their own staff to create new and innovative content.

Economics of Web Publishing

The Internet culture always has contended that content on the Web should be free. However, there are hard economic realities involved for those who want to maintain a site. These include costs for state-of-the-art hardware and software, Internet connection fees, and salaries for personnel with hard-to-find skills. Budd (2000) examined the various costs in some detail.

Think about how costs are recovered for printed journals. Subscription fees contribute little to the operating costs. Most of the financial support comes from advertising revenue. When advertisers place an advertisement in a printed journal, they estimate how many people "see" that page from verified numbers of subscribers. Whether people really "see" it is debatable. Many advertisers still are struggling with how to use the Web.

Several different approaches currently are being tried to recover costs of putting journals on-line. Some journals have a separate subscription to their on-line version. Some provide a pricing incentive to subscribe to both the print and on-line versions, and some provide access to the electronic version for "free" to print subscribers. Of course, nothing is free; someone pays. Sometimes, costs are recovered by adding to the subscription price or to organization dues when a publication is a benefit of membership.

Using Standardized General Markup Language (SGML), or a derivative such as Extensible Markup Language, is one step in significantly reducing costs. Simply defined, SGML is an international standard that provides the means for the description of encoded or marked up electronic text (Cover, 1999; Sperberg-McQueen & Burnard, 1996). Using SGML, text and images reside in a database. They then can be sent either to a composition house for printing or to the Web. The advantages of SGML are that it describes documents and categorizes parts of a document, and it is transportable from one hardware and software environment to another. Publishing companies are retooling to take advantage of SGML, but it requires some major changes in work flow and processes.

An initiative that may have significant impact on cost and availability of scholarly information on the Web is PubMed Central, a repository for life science research articles available on-line. PubMed Central, originally termed E-biomed, was proposed by Harold Varmus in 1999, while he was the Director of the National Institutes of Health (NIH). NIH considers this repository to be the initial site in an international system. PubMed Central archives, organizes, and distributes peer-reviewed reports from journals, as well as reports that have been screened but not formally peer reviewed. In addition, it coordinates with similar efforts to establish servers internationally, including those overseen by the European Molecular Biology Organization (NIH, 1999). Publishers, professional societies, and other groups independent of NIH have complete responsibility for the input to PubMed Central. Copyright resides with these groups or the authors themselves (NIH, 1999). NIH provides maintenance of the repository, including archiving content. There was considerable debate when the idea initially was proposed, with heated arguments both pro and con.

Stage 2: Trying New Things on the Web

Some of the resources on Web sites visited in this and other chapters are moving toward Stage 2 in Naisbitt's framework. They are implementing new ideas and are attempting to exploit the unique features of the new technology. Two specific instances of moving to Stage 2 are discussed here.

Writing in a Different Mode

The capabilities of the Web allow for exploration of new ways of structuring content. There is no need to follow a linear model in an interactive medium. The challenge is to write a cohesive, short article with embedded hyperlinks where content is explained in more detail. Murray (1997), a nursing colleague from the United Kingdom, has used this new structure for articles.

An on-line journal, *Kairos: A Journal for Teachers of Writing in Webbed Environments* (*http://english.ttu.edu/kairos/index.html*), deals specifically with the challenges of writing in hypertextual environments, primarily (but not solely) on the Web. The journal is designed as a peer-reviewed resource for teachers, researchers, and tutors of writing at the college and university level, including technical writing, professional communication, creative writing, composition, and literature.

Interactive Content With Multimedia Elements

On the Web, many media elements can be used by authors to further illustrate their content or provide an alternative presentation mode. For example, the *Internet Journal of Advanced Nursing Practice* (*http://www.ispub.com/journals/ijanp.htm*) contains audio and video files that demonstrate procedures.

A well-known instructional designer, Jonassen (1985), wrote an article that discussed 144 ways to vary an instructional event. Any given material can incorporate many instructional events. Which of the 144+ ways available on the Web should be chosen to deliver a given segment of the content:

- Text
- Hypertext
- Hypertext with graphics
- An animation
- Audio
- Video
- A three-dimensional model?

Although the strengths and weaknesses of an individual medium are known, when media are combined, the result is not just a combination of discrete elements but something new and different, which should do a better job of conveying the content than any of the elements could do alone. Multimedia has been used in computer products, mainly CD-ROM. But the same design, transferred to a different delivery system like the Web, changes it again. The new delivery system has intrinsic characteristics that may enhance or minimize the effectiveness of any media component. For example, current band width does not yet support high-quality, full-screen video delivery. Video clips must be short and can occupy only a portion of the screen, and motion often is "choppy." As band width increases, these limitations will be overcome.

Short quizzes with images began to appear early on some Web sites. Medscape, for example, provided a short patient history with accompanying ECG strips and microscopy slides as diagnostic challenges to physicians. To exploit the current capabilities of the Web, a team of nurses at Lippincott Williams & Wilkins designed an interactive case study experience. "Nursing Rounds" is a self-assessment CE offering based on Benner's (1982) "novice-to-expert" approach. Although the nurses who conceived of this idea immediately recognized the interactive potential, the concept was first incorporated into a print article with an accompanying test. When it migrated to NursingCenter.com, developers added a patient chart, a library with drug monographs, images, and links to other articles and Web sites. A database was created to collect answers to the multiple-choice questions and display the spread of responses, in Benner's novice-to-expert categories, from people who completed the offering. A forum also was created so that those who participated could discuss the case with the author. Unfortunately, only a few people availed themselves of this opportunity.

Therefore, an electronic article can evolve into an interactive case study. In this way, it appears more like something nurses see on a CD-ROM.

Another approach is the creation of a CE offering that begins with an article, but the answers to the test questions reside on another Web site. For example, an article on infection control might ask a question whose answer can be found on the Centers for Disease Control's Web site (*http://www.cdc.gov*). This approach exposes nurses to reputable Web sites that expand on the content of the article.

Before Moving to Stage 3: What Are Disadvantages and Risks?

The virtues of electronic publishing cannot be extolled without also pointing out the disadvantages. A book and journal are a known quantity. They have readily apparent beginning and ending points. They are self-contained and have well-understood conventions, such as tables of contents and indexes, which facilitate finding specific content.

The morphing boundaries of a Web site can be daunting to novice users. It can be disconcerting to find that by following a series of hyperlinks, the user has travelled well beyond the original Web site intended for access. Sparks (1999) and Ludwick and Glazer (2000) detailed some of the other disadvantages of on-line publishing, such as technical requirements (eg, need for computer, software, and modem) and the limited access resulting from these technical requirements. They also discussed the "unfriendliness" of some sites and the lack of technical standards. For example, files created for specific versions of browsers or plug-ins may look different when displayed in another browser, and certain parts of a Web page may not be displayed at all.

The most serious disadvantage is the lack of standards for archiving. The archiving dilemma, though, is not unsolvable. Standards can be established and responsibilities can be delegated to appropriate parties. These initiatives are important so that the valuable materials currently being created are not lost.

Because promotion and tenure needs drive many faculty to write journal articles, authors should take a moment to consider whether there are risks involved in publishing in an on-line–only journal and devoting time to developing an electronic product. There are always technophobes who are skeptical of anything new that involves technology that they do not understand. Those attitudes are changing quickly as the Web becomes ubiquitous. Fortunately, forward-thinking individuals recognize the issues and are examining and supporting electronic publishing efforts.

Stage 3: The Future

The print version of journals will continue to exist for some time, but printed journals will be forced to change as electronic delivery gains acceptance. Think about what happened to radio when television arrived. Previously, radio stations broadcasted a variety of different types of programs at different times of the day: regular news updates, soap operas in the morning, and drama and comedy entertainment at night. When television came along with its exciting visual attributes, radio did not disappear, but its position on the entertainment landscape changed. Radio stations became specialized. They now focus on one area, such as news or country music.

The opposite, though, may happen with printed journals. They may move away from a specialty focus to a more broad-based approach. If the nurse's clinical focus is cardiac care and the nurse wants to identify the latest treatment recommendations for an acute myocardial infarction, this information can be found easily through MEDLINE or another search engine. Health care news and its implications for nursing practice, though, are not found in a MEDLINE search. A journal that provides a clinical focus, job opportunities, news, and issues might be useful because the editors already would have distilled the important information about what is happening in that field. Delivering this type of broad focus will be accommodated on the Web in the future, but for now, the ability to have content bundled in an attractive print format has its own gestalt, in addition to providing a level of comfort and familiarity.

Customized Subscriptions

What will the Stage 3 of electronic publishing look like? First, subscriptions may be customized. The nurse may be able to obtain electronic subscriptions of full-text articles from many journals, which are generated according to a user profile provided by the nurse. If the nurse's primary clinical focus is cardiac care and the nurse currently is working in administration in a long-term care facility, the nurse could ask for articles or abstracts on clinical cardiac topics, administration, and issues in long-term care. It may be possible to specify which articles should be full text and which should be abstracts. If the abstracts are of interest, full text of the article would be available with a quick click, probably for an additional fee.

Multimedia Articles

Second, as band width increases, the ability to add multimedia elements to articles and other forms of information will evolve. These will not have a print equivalent. Instead, they will use pictures, graphics, animation, sound, and video files to explain and illustrate beyond the capabilities of print. This will require authors to work with others to create and deliver content.

Multimedia Delivery System

Third, in addition to multimedia articles, the Web also will be a multimedia delivery system for educational and informational products of all kinds. Currently, the cost of developing these products—typically on CD-ROM—has demanded that they be sold at a high price; thus, they are purchased mostly by institutions. If the Web can promote and deliver these products to individuals, an increased volume of sales, coupled with savings in promotion and shipping costs, can make them affordable to individuals.

COPYRIGHT AND ETHICS

The electronic world makes it easy to cut and paste from the Web to the author's own word processor. When doing this, authors need to be careful to include the source. Plagiarism always has existed, but the electronic world makes it easier. Sometimes, committing plagiarism is unintentional. Users copy or cut and paste something found on the Web that stimulates a thought or confirms their own beliefs. If prospective authors do not document the source immediately, when they return to that notation later, perhaps to write an article, they may think that the note was their own idea. Authors always must document the source at the time the information is gathered.

The practice of assigning copyright to a publisher appears to be continuing in the on-line world. For example, the OJNI manuscript guidelines indicate that the author needs to assign the copyright to OJNI. *Kairos* (1999) takes a modified approach and requires the right to publish, distribute, archive, and make an article permanently retrievable electronically, but authors retain their copyright. The *Kairos* policy is to allow authors to republish the information as long as they acknowledge *Kairos* as the original site of publication.

Assigning copyright to a publisher is a practice that is widely misunderstood. Assigning copyright puts the onus of protecting an author's work on the publishing company.

 ## SOME FINAL THOUGHTS

The future of electronic publishing and information delivery on the Web requires new ways of thinking and doing. It will be a team approach because many different skills are required to deliver the interactive product. Some ideas will spark, then die. Some good ideas will whither because of social or economic forces. One recent idea was to include raw research data with the on-line published research findings; others could build on the data, add to the sample, and reanalyze the data. This effort failed, though, because researchers were not willing to release their raw data. Other new ideas and applications, however, will evolve and survive as the possibilities of the new electronic techno-tools are realized.

Jones and Cook (2000) explored the question of whether electronic journals are a paradigm shift. They concluded that until electronic journals move beyond their current two-dimensional boundaries, they are only a different delivery mode. As people depend more on the Web as a source of information, it will change individuals and society as a whole.

Earlier, McLuhan (1964) said that technology changes us. He believed that form was more important than content. In other words, the fact that we have technology such as telephones, computers, and the Web is more important in shaping us than anything we say on the phone, any software that we use, or any information that we find on the Web. McLuhan believed that media influenced us by emphasizing certain senses at the expense of others. Print, for example, emphasizes the visual and fosters linear thought patterns. If McLuhan is correct, then nonsequential hypermedia applications should foster a change in the direction of more creative, mosaic thinking.

McLuhan also believed that media change us by altering social arrangements among people, causing shifts in images of ourselves and our roles in society. For example, the move from an oral to a print society fostered new attitudes and feelings about privacy and individualism. According to McLuhan, reading requires quiet and privacy, and this aspect of print media fostered the emergence of feelings about the importance of individuality in contrast to the "good of the group" philosophy that had previously prevailed.

If he is right, will the need to work cooperatively to produce multimedia experiences for electronic publishing cause us to value cooperative group work over individuality? Or will it be offset by increased time working and learning at home with less face-to-face interpersonal and group participation as part of our day? The implications for us as individuals and for our society as a whole are enormous and require that careful attention be paid to the influence of this fast-paced technology thrust on us as the new millennium unfolds.

SUMMARY

The Internet and the World Wide Web mark the beginning of an era that is changing the world. In the arena of electronic publication, the Web opens up possibilities for greater exposure and dissemination of articles and information. It allows for collaborative workspace and can accommodate different formats for delivering content.

When an article is accepted for publication, the author may find it published on the Web before or after it appears in the printed journal. Some authors may decide to submit an article to an on-line–only journal.

Early in Web history, journals began to appear on the Web that never existed in print format. There are several advantages to publishing directly to the Web: articles can be published more quickly, there is no need to wait, and there are no page or space restrictions. Publication on the Web makes articles accessible worldwide. Search engines automatically add the publication to their databases, and translation software can make the information available in other languages. On-line nursing journals already are available, and their development is likely to continue.

'Zines are different from on-line journals. Some are delivered by e-mail, some are posted on the Web, and some come in both forms. They generally are not peer reviewed as are on-line journals. Most 'zines contain what's new–type features rather than scholarly information.

Portals refer to Web sites offering a broad array of resources and services. Generally, a portal has a significant amount of content and also acts as a point of access to content on other Web sites of interest to their users. Portals contain community-building areas, such as forums and chat discussions.

The capabilities of the Web allow for exploration of new ways of structuring content. There is no need to follow a linear model in an interactive medium. The challenge is to write a cohesive, short article with embedded hyperlinks, where content is explained in more detail. Many media elements can be used by authors to further illustrate their content or provide an alternative presentation mode.

Electronic publishing provides many new opportunities for nursing authors. The Internet and the Web mark the beginning of an era that is changing the way individuals communicate knowledge and new ideas.

REFERENCES

Benner, P. (1982). From novice to expert. *American Journal of Nursing, 82*(3), 402–407.

Budd, K.W. (2000). The economic of electronic journals. *Online Journal of Issues in Nursing.* [On-line]. Available: *http://nursingworld.org/ojin/topic11/tpc11_3.htm.* Accessed July 9, 2000.

Cover, R. (1999). SGML: General introductions and overviews. OASIS: The XML cover pages. [On-line]. Available: *http://www.oasis-open.org/cover/general.html.* Accessed April 4, 2000.

Jonassen, D.H. (1985). Interactive lesson designs: A taxonomy. *Educational Technology, 25*(6), 7–17.

Jones, S.L., & Cook, C.B. (2000). Electronic journals: Are they a paradigm shift? *Online Journal of Issues in Nursing.* [On-line]. Available: *http://www.nursingworld.org/ojin/topic11/tpc11_1.htm.* Accessed April 4, 2000.

Kairos. (1999). Submissions. [On-line]. Available: *http://english.ttu.edu/kairos.* Accessed July 9, 2000.

Ludwick. R., & Glazer G. (2000). Electronic publishing: The movement from print to digital publication. *Online Journal of Issues in Nursing.* [On-line]. Available: *http:www.ana.org/ojin/topic11/tpc11_2.htm.* Accessed April 2, 2000.

McLuhan, M. (1964). *Understanding media: The extensions of man.* New York: McGraw-Hill.

Murray, P.J. (1997). A rose by any other name. *CMC Magazine.* [On-line]. Available: *http://www.december.com/cmc/mag/1997/jan/murray.html.* Accessed April 4, 2000.

Murray, P.J., & Anthony, D.M. (1999). Current and future models for nursing e-journals: Making the most of the webs' potential. *International Journal of Medical Informatics, 53,* 151–161.

Naisbitt, J. (1991). *Megatrends.* New York: Warner Books.

National Institutes of Health. (1999). PubMed Central: An NIH-Operated Site for Electronic Distribution of Life Sciences Research Reports. [On-line]. Available: *http://www.nih.gov/about/director/pubmedcentral/pubmedcentral.htm.* Accessed July 3, 2000.

Online Journal of Nursing Informatics (OJNI). (1999). Contributor's guidelines. [On-line]. Available: *http://milkman.cac.psu.edu/dxm12/OJNI.html.* Accessed July 9, 2000.

Sparks, S. (1999). Electronic publishing and nursing research. *Nursing Research, 48*(1), 50–54.

Sperberg-McQueen, C.M., & Burnard, L. (Eds.). (1996). A gentle introduction to SGML: Guidelines for electronic text encoding and interchange (TEI P3). [On-line]. Available: *http://www-tel.ulc.edu/org/tei/sgml/teip3sg/SG.htm.* Accessed April 3, 2000.

Strom, D. (1996). Lessons learned from becoming a self-publisher on the web. *CMC Magazine.* [On-line]. Available: *http://www.december.com/cmc/mag/1996/may/strom.html.* Accessed April 4, 2000.

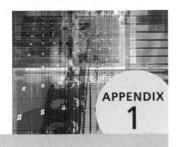

Manuscript	Typeset	Definition
ANCOVA	ANCOVA	Analysis of covariance
ANOVA	ANOVA	Analysis of variance (univariate)
d	d	Cohen's measure of effect size
d'	d'	(d prime) measure of sensitivity
D	D	Used in Kolmogorov–Smirnov test
f	f	Frequency
f_e	f_e	Expected frequency
F	F	Fisher's F ratio
F_{max}	F_{max}	Hartley's test of variance homogeneity
H	H	Used in Kruskal–Wallis test; also used to mean *hypothesis*
H_0	H_0	Null hypothesis under test
H_1	H_1	Alternative hypothesis
HSD	HSD	Tukey's honestly significant difference (also referred to as the Tukey a procedure)
k	k	Coefficient of alienation
k^2	k^2	Coefficient of nondetermination
K-R 20	K-R 20	Kuder–Richardson formula
LR	LR	Likelihood ratio (used with some chi-squares)
LSD	LSD	Fisher's least significant difference
M	M	Mean (arithmetic average)
MANOVA	MANOVA	Multivariate analysis of variance
Mdn	Mdn	Median

(table continues)

Manuscript	*Typeset*	*Definition*
mle	*mle*	Maximum likelihood estimate (used with programs such as LISREL)
mode	mode	Most frequently occurring score
MS	*MS*	Mean square
MSE	*MSE*	Mean square error
n	*n*	Number in a subsample
N	*N*	Total number in a sample
ns	*ns*	Nonsignificant
p	*p*	Probability; also the success probability of a binomial variable
P	*P*	Percentage, percentile
pr	*pr*	Partial correlation
q	*q*	$1 - p$ for a binomial variable
Q	*Q*	Quartile (also used in Cochran's test)
r	*r*	Pearson product–moment correlation
r^2	r^2	Pearson product–moment correlation squared; coefficient of determination
r_b	r_b	Biserial correlation
r_k	r_k	Reliability of mean *k* judges' ratings
r_1	r_1	Estimated reliability of the typical judge
r_{pb}	r_{pb}	Point-biserial correlation
r_s	r_s	Spearman rank correlation coefficient (formerly rho [ρ])
R	*R*	Multiple correlation; also composite rank, a significance test
R^2	R^2	Multiple correlation squared; measure of strength of relationship
SD	*SD*	Standard deviation
SE	*SE*	Standard error
SEM	*SEM*	Standard error of measurement
sr	*sr*	Semipartial correlation

Manuscript	Typeset	Definition
$\underline{SS}$	SS	Sum of squares
$\underline{t}$	t	Computed value of t test
$\underline{T}$	T	Computed value of Wilcoxon's or McCall's test
$\underline{T}^2$	T^2	Computed value of Hotelling's test
Tukey $\underline{a}$	Tukey a	Tukey's HSD procedure
$\underline{U}$	U	Computed value of Mann–Whitney test
$\underline{V}$	V	Cramér's statistic for contingency tables; Pillai–Bartlett multivariate criterion
$\underline{W}$	W	Kendall's coefficient of concordance
$\underline{x}$	x	Abscissa (horizontal axis in graph)
$\underline{y}$	y	Ordinate (vertical axis in graph)
$\underline{z}$	z	A standard score; difference between one value in a distribution and the mean of the distribution divided by the SD
$\lvert \underline{a} \rvert$	$\lvert a \rvert$	Absolute value of a
α	α	Alpha; probability of a Type I error; Cronbach's index of internal consistency
β	β	Beta; probability of a Type II error ($1 - \beta$ is statistical power); standardized multiple regression coefficient
γ	γ	Gamma; Goodman–Kruskal's index of relationship
Δ	Δ	Delta (cap); increment of change
η^2	η^2	Eta squared; measure of strength of relationship
θ	Θ	Theta (cap); Roy's multivariate criterion

Manuscript	Typeset	Definition
λ	λ	Lambda; Goodman–Kruskal's measure of predictability
Λ	Λ	Lambda (cap); Wilks's multivariate criterion
ν	ν	Nu; degrees of freedom
ρ_I	ρ_I	Rho (with subscript); intraclass correlation coefficient
Σ	Σ	Sigma (cap); sum or summation
τ	τ	Tau; Kendall's rank correlation coefficient; also Hotelling's multivariate trace criterion
ϕ	ϕ	Phi; measure of association for a contingency table; also a parameter used in determining sample size or statistical power
ϕ^2	ϕ^2	Phi squared; proportion of variance accounted for in a 2×2 contingency table
χ^2	χ^2	Computed value of a chi-square test
Ψ	Ψ	Psi; a statistical comparison
ω^2	ω^2	Omega squared; measure of strength of relationship
$\wedge$	$\wedge$	(caret) when above a Greek letter (or parameter), indicates an estimate (or statistic)

Note. Greek symbols are lowercase unless noted otherwise.

PROOFREADERS' MARKS

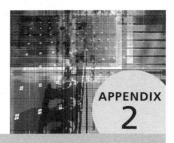

Proofreaders' Marks

OPERATIONAL SIGNS

Mark	Meaning
ℛ	Delete
⊂	Close up; delete space
ℛ̃	Delete and close up (use only when deleting letters *within* a word)
stet	Let it stand
#	Insert space
eq #	Make space between words equal; make space between lines equal
hr #	Insert hair space
ls	Letterspace
¶	Begin new paragraph
☐	Indent type one em from left or right
⊐	Move right
⊏	Move left
⊐⊏	Center
⊓	Move up
⊔	Move down
fl	Flush left
fr	Flush right
=	Straighten type; align horizontally
‖	Align vertically
tr	Transpose
sp	Spell out

TYPOGRAPHICAL SIGNS

Mark	Meaning
ital	Set in italic type
rom	Set in roman type
bf	Set in boldface type
lc	Set in lowercase
caps	Set in capital letters
sc	Set in small capitals
wf	Wrong font; set in correct type
X	Check type image; remove blemish
V	Insert here *or* make superscript
Λ	Insert here *or* make subscript

PUNCTUATION MARKS

Mark	Meaning
⌃	Insert comma
⌄ ⌄	Insert apostrophe *or* single quotation mark
⌄⌄ ⌄⌄	Insert quotation marks
⊙	Insert period
set ?	Insert question mark
;/	Insert semicolon
⌃ or :/	Insert colon
=	Insert hyphen
M	Insert em dash
N	Insert en dash
⊏/ᵬor (/)	Insert parentheses

299

] Authors As Proofreaders [

"I don't care what kind of type you use for my book," said a myopic author to the publisher, but please print the galley proofs in large type. Perhaps in the future such a request will not sound so ridiculous to those familar with the printing process. today, however, type once set is not reset exept to correct errors. Proofreading is an Art and a craft. All authors should know the rudiaments thereof, though no proof-reader expects them to be masters of it. Watch proof-reader expects them to be masters of it. Watch not only for misspelled or incorrect works (often a most illusive error, but also for misplace dspaces, "unclose" quotation marks and parenthesis, and impoper paragraphing; and learn to recognize the difference between an em dash—used to separate an interjectional part of a sentence—and an en dash used commonly between continuing numbers, e.g., pp. 5–10; a.d. 1165 70) and the word dividing hyphen. Whatever is underlined in a MS. should of course, be italicized in print. Two lines drawn beneath letters or words indicate that these are to be reset in small capitals three lines indicate full capitals To find the errors overlooked by the proof-reader is the author's first problem in proof reading. The secyond problem is to make corrections using the marks and symbols, devized by proffesional proof-readers, that any trained typesetter will understand. The third—and most difficult problem for authors proofreading their own works is to resist the temptation to rewrite in proofs.

Manuscript editor

1. Type may be reduced in size, or enlarged photographically when a book is printed by offset.

From *The Chicago Manual of Style* (14th ed.). (1993). Chicago: The University of Chicago Press, pp. 112–113. Reprinted by permission of the University of Chicago Press. © 1993 by the University of Chicago.

INDEX

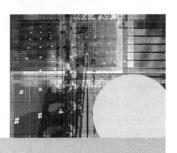

Note: Page numbers followed by *f* indicate figures; those followed by *t*
indicate tables; those followed by *d* indicate displays.